STAY FOREVER YOUNG

How to Prolong Youth, Health and Vitality with Bio-identical Hormones

By Greg Brannon, M.D.

© 2018 Greg Brannon, M.D. and The Youth Institute

ISBN-13: 9781727213676

ISBN-10: 172721367X

Medical Disclaimer:

The information, ideas, and suggestions in this book are not intended as a substitute for professional medical advice. The following text is for general information only. It contains the opinions and ideas of the author. This information is not intended to diagnose or treat any disease. Before following any suggestions contained in this book, you should consult your personal physician. Extensive research has been conducted and careful attention has been paid to insure the accuracy of the information herein, however, neither the author nor the publisher shall be liable or responsible for any loss, damage, or health consequence allegedly arising as a result of your use or application of any information or suggestions in this book.

Table of Contents

Dedication

First and foremost,

To my best friend and the biggest supporter of my life,

my wife, Jody.

I also want to dedicate this book to future knowledge-seekers.

*Remember: **Knowledge is power!***

Don't be afraid to question everything.

May this book cause you to study more deeply,

research more thoroughly, and push harder for the truth.

Liberty always requires responsibility.

Foreward by Charles Rizzuto, M.D.

As an anesthesiologist, I am an expert in human physiology and the pharmaceuticals that are available to modern medicine. I safely navigate patients through complex procedures, keeping their bodies in perfect homeostasis for the duration of the surgery. I care for patients with a wide range of medical conditions. Their health is affected by their lifestyle, genetics, environmental exposures, and the process of aging.

Dr. Greg Brannon is the Medical Director at The Youth Institute in Cary, North Carolina and has recently opened several other clinics in North Carolina as well. As an expert in his field, Dr. Brannon maintains that today, many of the common changes we see as one ages are not normal. These changes are mostly attributed to decreasing levels of hormones.

Dr. Brannon, a dear friend of mine for over 30 years, clearly explains how these changes occur in both men and women. As an OB-GYN for over 25 years, he is an expert in the hormonal changes that occur throughout one's lifetime. Dr. Brannon graduated from the University of Southern California in 1982. He went on to graduate from The University of Health and Science Chicago Medical School in 1988 and completed his residency in OB-GYN at the University of Southern California Women's Hospital in 1992. He served as a Clinical Assistant Professor at the University of North Carolina School of Medicine, and has been in private practice in the Raleigh-Durham area since 1993. Dr. Brannon lives in North Carolina with his lovely wife Jody, where they have raised 7 children.

In the pages that follow, Dr. Brannon explores the common changes we experience with aging. He emphasizes that "what is common is not necessarily normal." He describes how hormones work, and that as we age, the levels of important hormones decrease. He explains the various causes of these decreases. He describes what happens to the body as we correct these deficiencies with bio-identical hormone replacement therapy (BHRT). He explains how synthetic hormone replacement differs from BHRT. While acknowledging the controversies surrounding replacement therapy, he cites multiple research articles to support the superiority of this methodology. He explains the advantages of pellet placement therapy over other delivery methods, detailing how the procedure is performed, and why it is the preferred method of hormone administration for producing a smoother onset and longer steady state of blood level concentrations. His many success stories of patients whose lives have been greatly improved illustrate how Dr. Brannon puts his talent and great knowledge to work. Finally, he concludes by explaining how one can easily get started with bio-identical hormone replacement.

Introduction by Greg Brannon, M.D.

Knowledge is power.

When you have knowledge about how your body works and how to get your life back, you have *power.*

How much do you know about how your body functions? How in-tune are you with what's going on inside of you? Do you know the basic principles of hormones and how they relate to your health?

You are about to discover some of the best research available about how to maintain maximum health and vitality as you age – through Bio-identical Hormone Replacement Therapy (BHRT).

BHRT is not new. It has been around a long time - since the 1930s. Those early researchers and proponents discovered something very profound: in order to "reverse aging," you have to recreate the "chemistry of youth" inside the human body. That perfect chemistry is simply a matter of sufficient levels of hormones so that the body can perform all of its various functions with ease.

The goal of this book is to illustrate how balanced and abundant levels of hormones facilitate prime health optimization.

A wise man once said, "We are not conscious of the three greatest blessings in life: health, youth, and freedom, while we possess them, but only after we have lost them." [i]

One thing many people have lost today is the blessing of good health. Our bodies have changed. Many are facing depression, low energy, poor focus, low libido, and a myriad of other diseases and symptoms. People are not aging gracefully anymore. And it's not just those in their 40s and older. I'm frequently seeing men and women in their 20s with hormone deficiencies.

In the pages that follow, I hope to make you aware of the overwhelming amount of research that illustrates the positive effects of bio-identical hormone replacement therapy. When our hormone levels return to normal – to where they *should be* – our bodies will be strengthened and have the best chance of aging gracefully and staying healthy and robust.

Everything I teach is backed up by medical research, white papers, scientific studies, and my own experience. I will mention some of the extensive documented research periodically. However, my intent is that this introductory book be a quick and easy read for those seeking a brief overview on BHRT. For more detailed and extensive scientific evidence, I invite you to visit our website:

youthinstitutebhrt.com

I understand that there is a degree of controversy over hormone replacement therapy. There are opinions on each side, and it is up to you to do your own research and come to your own conclusions about what is best for you.

My Personal Motivation

My firm belief that bio-identical hormones are the key to vibrant health comes from personal experience. Not only did I devote myself to many years of study, reading research papers, and years of clinical practice, but I am also currently receiving bio-identical hormone treatments myself, and I have experienced a profound personal transformation. I want others to have the opportunity to feel as good as I do, physically and mentally. My beautiful wife Jody, who is the love of my life and the mother of my seven children, is also currently receiving bio-identical hormone replacement therapy, which should tell you how much I trust and believe in the safety and effectiveness of these treatments.

Those who know me well know that I have always followed a path of questioning everything. During my residency at USC Women's hospital, I was trained in the Socratic method, which ingrained in me a lifelong habit of asking penetrating questions. Instead of simply researching which drugs are being prescribed for patients who are sick, I want to know first, *"Why* are we so sick, as a population?" "Why are there more chronic diseases than ever?" "Why is there such a long list of health complications today that we have not seen in the past?"

After asking those questions, I research deeply and thoroughly for the answers so that I can find the real *cause*. In finding the *cause* of what ails us, we will find the best *cure*. As a practicing OB/GYN for the last 27 years, I have had firsthand personal relationships with many of my patients. I know them well and have delivered their babies in most cases. I care deeply about their long-term health, well-being and happiness and about the lives of their families. In everything I do, I'm looking for answers that will help the individual. And I'm on a quest to help each one of my patients according to his or her health-related needs and wants. I believe the individual should be the final authority over his or her personal health care.

Let's Begin the Conversation

I'd like everyone reading this book to feel as though they are having a frank and informative one-on-one conversation with me. Imagine coming into my office and sitting down. You have my undivided attention. And you've come prepared with a list of questions about bio-identical hormone treatment. This book contains my honest, straightforward answers to the most often-asked questions on the subject.

I'll explain why the problem of decreasing hormone levels is affecting the general population physically. I'll explain how, when hormone levels are optimized, the body is better protected against aging, disease, injuries, and fatigue.

I will explain how hormones work. I will discuss 6 causes for lower hormone levels among men and women today, and I'll delve into some of the medical studies and literature that reveal the benefits of proper hormone treatment.

I will detail the difference between synthetic hormone treatments and their dangers, and bio-identical hormone treatments, and their benefits. I will illustrate how bio-identical hormone replacement therapy (BHRT) restores deficient hormones, repairs the body on a cellular level, improves overall health, and ultimately revitalizes the well-being of the individual.

Finally, I will discuss the process of receiving BHRT and talk about how simple it is to get started.

In the final chapter, I have also included a short reading list of five foundational books that I believe you will find helpful as you do your own investigation.

For practical reasons, my intention is that this small handbook serves as a pared-down, factual guide to beginning bio-identical hormone replacement therapy at The Youth Institute.

How The Youth Institute Began

The Youth Institute was established in Cary, North Carolina in March of 2012. To date, we have treated over 3,000 patients, both men and women. I have patients as young as 18 and, at this point, the oldest is 86. We have recently opened three new locations – in Wake Forest, Wilmington, and Southern Pines/Pinehurst – and more locations are on the way!

I am so excited about BHRT, and to tell you about this treatment. My discovery of bio-identical hormones is what has caused me to enter a second career, medically speaking. I have been an OB/GYN doctor for the last 27 years. Earlier in my career, I prescribed synthetic hormones for women entering menopause. I didn't know any better. It's what I had been taught in medical school, residency, and post-residency training. I was taught that there was no difference between the way synthetic hormones and bio-identical hormones work in our bodies. Boy, was I wrong!

About 10 years ago, I was introduced to bio-identical hormone replacement therapy through a friend who had started the treatment himself. My first reaction was to say, "Hey buddy, you're going to kill yourself. That stuff causes prostate cancer!"

To be honest, it was my own arrogance and ignorance that caused me to be closed-minded on this subject. I simply had not educated myself on the differences between bio-identicals vs. synthetics.

Fortunately, I've always been a science nerd. I've always read and studied inquisitively. And the changes in my friend's life intrigued me, so I began doing my own research and study. I not only came to the conclusion that BHRT was effective, but *essential* for healthy aging. So, I became a patient as well. I know first-hand the results of this treatment. I believe in it with all my heart, and I'm going to share it with you.

Health Freedom

As Americans, we have a right to liberty and freedom – political, religious, and medical freedom. There are those who would like to restrict your access to safe, natural, alternative therapies such as bio-identical hormones. The more people know the truth about what options are available to them, the more likely it will be that these therapies will remain accessible to the general public.

"If people let the government decide what foods they eat and what medicines they take, their bodies will soon be in as sorry a state as are the souls of those who live under tyranny."

~ Thomas Jefferson[ii]

Come join me in this journey and let me convince you why bio-identical hormones are for you. Let me take you back to the basics of hormonal balance, drawing on thousands of research papers and studies which demonstrate that bio-identical hormones are safe, proven, and effective.

Chapter 1 – We All Want to Stay "Forever Young"

As far back as we can remember in human history, man searched and hoped for and sought after an elusive "Fountain of Youth." There are myths and stories about the quest for Eternal Youth. Books and poems and countless songs have been written on the subject. Every new diet, weight loss aid, beauty product or surgical procedure promises to make us "look younger." Our culture most certainly has an obsession with looking young, feeling young, and staying young.

And with good reason! The health, energy, vitality and beauty we enjoy in our youth is something we don't fully appreciate until we start to lose it. We all want to feel as good as we did when we were ages 20 to 30. What many people do not realize is that the invincible way we felt during that decade of life was due to an abundance of magical chemical messengers inside our bodies called hormones. And that simply restoring that abundance can restore our "youth" to a surprising extent.

Now, a certain degree of aging is inevitable. We cannot expect to have a "babyface," boundless energy, and a child's spirit forever. We can, however, hold onto a younger, fresher appearance, an active lifestyle, and many of the cherished qualities and sensations of being young longer than we ever thought possible.

After 7 years of administering bio-identical hormones to thousands of surprised and happy patients, I can honestly say that bio-identical pellet therapy is the *closest thing to the Fountain of Youth* available to us right here and now, in the 21st century.

13

"Aging Early" Has Become Acceptable

The medical community and today's society are **perpetuating a myth** that the following are "normal" occurrences due to aging:

- It is "normal" to have a decreased libido as we age.

- It is "normal" for young women to lose interest sexually, to suffer from vaginal dryness, and to experience unexplained mood swings.

- It is "normal" for young women to have PMS, hot flashes, and night sweats.

- It is "normal" that our current population has an ever-increasing number of people being diagnosed with dementia, Alzheimer's, and diabetes.

- It is "normal" to experience significant weight gain as you age and to have difficulty losing that weight, no matter how much you diet or exercise.

- It is "normal" for men to have an absence of nighttime erections and to have difficulty maintaining a strong erection during intercourse.

- It is "normal" for middle-aged men to lose muscle mass, muscle tone, and to experience weight gain, especially around the waist.

- It is "normal" for young couples, 25 - 35 years of age, to only have sexual intimacy once or twice every few months.

- It is "normal" for people of any age to be on 3 or 4 anti-depressants at a time.

These things have become acceptable, and it's a shame that we as a society do not question these occurrences. They may be common, but they are certainly not normal.

"Common" is not necessarily synonymous with "normal."

The good news is that all of these problems can be addressed and remedied.

Over the last 5 decades, our society has seen an alarming increase in the onslaught and intensity of diseases that we have accepted as normal. We have a generation of adults that are suffering in great numbers from diseases that the previous generation experienced in small numbers. Fifty years ago, conditions such as diabetes, dementia and Alzheimer's were far less prevalent.[iii] Cardiovascular disease too has skyrocketed.[iv] Again, just because the current situation is common, that does not mean that it's normal.

What is normal for the human body is a perfect state of health, not a state of disease. Just because so many people in our society are ill doesn't mean that we were designed to live in a perpetual state of sickness.

Have you ever stopped to consider that getting older does not have to mean falling apart?

We Are Losing Hormones as We Age

Every one of us longs for health and vitality. We're aware, in this "mega-information era" that it's common for men and women to experience decreasing hormone levels as they age, resulting in diminished energy and focus, among other things.

When scientists were seeking to harness nuclear energy, they realized if they fired a neutron of uranium against other uranium atoms, they could create an unbelievably powerful nuclear reaction. This was the method used to create the atomic bomb. The neutrons released when the atoms split would, in turn, strike and split other atoms. Think

15

about that. Scientists discovered and harnessed a power source of energy (sometimes used for good, sometimes for evil) that was revolutionary.

This same type of reaction happens in your body and mine. Testosterone starts a chain reaction in our bodies. It replenishes our cells, which, in turn, strengthens our organs and systems. Through bio-identical hormone replacement therapy or "BHRT," science has identified an effective and safe way to replenish the power source in our bodies.

Did you get that?

No longer must we be resigned to living with the debilitating effects of low hormone levels. No longer do we have to suffer from diseases without having the natural resources and power to fight those diseases. It is a revolutionary concept that has changed the lives of thousands of people. And it can change yours. It can help you get your "youth" back.

Now, let me be clear: BHRT is not a panacea. It is not a magic wand that can be waved over your body so you will never be sick again. But when your hormone levels return to their ideal levels – to where they *should* be – your body will be strengthened, and you will have the very best chance of aging gracefully, and staying healthy and strong.

Throughout this book, I am going to be very practical. I want to answer the questions that most people, and probably you, are asking. I will delve into the science behind bio-identicals only to the extent that it helps answer the questions you may have. To learn more, visit our website to find extensive resources and scientific research papers.

At any time, you may go to **youthinstitutebhrt.com** to find hundreds of articles and/or details about becoming a patient at The Youth Institute.

Chapter 2 – The Importance of Hormones

Our bodies are unique and wonderfully designed. They have been created to function in perfect hormonal balance. When our bodies experience that divine equilibrium, the result is health and fitness. But when our hormones are out of whack, the results can be disastrous.

Hormones are chemical messengers created by the body to transfer information from one set of cells to another. As they are released into the bloodstream, they coordinate and control the various functions of the body to maintain health and stability.

The endocrine system in your body is made up of glands that produce and secrete hormones to regulate the activity of cells or organs. Hormones regulate the body's growth, metabolism, sexual development and function. When our hormone levels drop, becoming imbalanced, our health is affected.

Testosterone is the chemical that enables every single cell in your body make protein. This DNA cell replication is called transcription. What are you made up of? Cells and cellular structures. When your cells are weak, your organs and systems are weak, and YOU become weak.

Hormones are designed to strengthen our bodies at the cellular level. Therefore, we must get to the root causes to find out what goes wrong when hormone levels drop.

Let's talk a little science for a moment …

Epigenetics

Epigenetics is the study of changes in organisms caused by modification of gene expression rather than an alteration of the genetic code itself. In the last 10 years, we've discovered that how we live, what we eat, how much stress we deal with, and various other factors influence our DNA expression throughout our lifetimes. In other words, your DNA is not something static that you inherit from your parents and then, you're stuck with it. It is constantly changing either for the better or worse, according to how you live. Your very DNA structure is affected by environmental factors, diet, viruses, and even vaccines. You can, to a large extent, control the expression of your genes. You are not necessarily doomed to get cancer or Parkinson's or whatever other hereditary illnesses may run in your family. If you take care of yourself, you can literally change your own biological "destiny."[v]

EDCs

In 2007, a study was published in The Journal of Endocrinology and Metabolism which concluded that American men are experiencing a substantial population-wide decrease in testosterone serum levels, due to compromised health and/or environmental factors.[vi] The findings prove that male testosterone levels have decreased every decade for the last 60 years. Why is this? The number one cause is **Endocrine-Disrupting Chemicals** (EDCs), also known as "estrogen mimickers." These chemicals influence the structure of sex hormones in our bodies. Please note: The purpose of sex hormones in your body is by no means limited to sex. Sex hormones control the majority of bodily functions; everything from your appetite, to your energy level, to your emotions, to your ability to heal, is the result of a properly functioning endocrine system. Hormonal balance creates a strong foundation for your health; in the same way that a brick house is strong because it's made out of bricks. A backbone of the 27-carbon structure in your body is cholesterol. From that cholesterol is formed your cortisol, your testosterone, your estrogen, your progesterone, and all the precursors to that.

Unfortunately, endocrine-disrupting chemicals are found *everywhere*: in plastics, pesticides, heavy metals, food additives, cleaning products, cash register receipts, and personal care products, just to name a few. When these endocrine-disrupting chemicals enter our bloodstreams, either orally or transdermally (absorbed through the skin), our very structures are compromised. Why? These estrogen mimickers "hide" in various places in our bodies. They affect your overall physiology: the hypothalamus, the pituitary gland, the testes, ovaries, and adrenal glands. EDCs are associated with altered reproductive function in both sexes, abnormal growth phenomena and neurocognitive problems in children, breast cancer, and compromised immune systems.[vii]

What does this mean?

Let's go back to our brick house analogy. The smallest structure in your body is a cell. Cells group together to make up your internal organs. And those organs group together to make up systems in your body. A brick house is made of ... bricks! But you need something to hold the bricks together. If you simply stack those bricks together, one on top of another, to form a wall, it will be a very unstable wall. Bricks need mortar to hold them together. The bricks are strong, only to the extent that they can hold together. **What mortar does for bricks, hormones do for the cells.** It strengthens them and helps them function efficiently and effectively as a group.

Human Physiology 101

To understand the implications of low hormone levels, it is necessary to comprehend some basic facts about human physiology and how hormones work.

Testosterone

Your DNA is the blueprint that makes cellular structures. Proteins are actually created from DNA. Before a double-stranded DNA helix is turned into a protein, it first goes through a process called "translation," and then, "transcription." Testosterone bypasses the cellular membrane and goes into the nucleus membrane, diffuses there and actually bonds to the DNA to turn on the DNA groups that form proteins. In short, testosterone is the gasoline that fuels your body's engine. Testosterone converts into both estradiol and into DHT (which is 10 times more potent than testosterone). All three of these hormones enter the blood system and are distributed throughout our bodies.

The diagram on the following page shows how hormones enter the blood stream and travel throughout your system. These chemical messengers coordinate complex processes like growth, metabolism, and fertility. The key point to understand is that hormones affect every cell in our bodies.

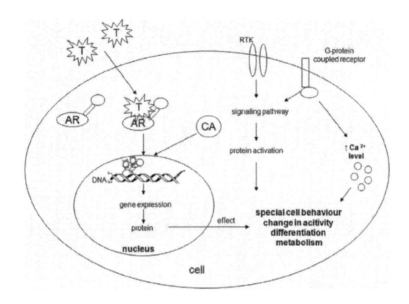

Progesterone

Many people think of progesterone as the "pregnancy hormone," and believe it only exists in females. But did you know that men produce progesterone too? Progesterone is a precursor to testosterone, and helps keep estrogen levels in check in the male body.

In the female body, progesterone is equally important, if not more so. Research shows that progesterone is important for breast health, cardiovascular health, nervous system health, and proper brain function.[viii] In women, this hormone is highest around post-ovulation times. In fact, women tend to feel their best during the second half of their monthly cycle, because that's when their progesterone level is at its highest. My goal is always to make sure that women have neither too much nor too little of this hormone. Progesterone levels can vary between 0 and 30 ng/ml, and I want to find the optimal levels for each woman.

FSH

Both men and women produce a chemical called FSH, or Follicle Stimulating Hormone in the pituitary gland. In women, this hormone stimulates the growth of ovarian follicles in the ovaries and increases estradiol production. In men, FSH stimulates sperm production in the testes. For menopausal women, it's important to monitor FSH and to replace estrogen. What I look for specifically is making sure FSH levels do not go above 20 mIU/ml. The higher that number goes, the more women will experience menopausal symptoms, like hot flashes, vaginal dryness, and sudden perspiration. So, as I monitor the blood labs, I can watch for those symptoms.

BHRT Replaces, Repairs, Restores, and Revitalizes!

Hormone Replacement Therapy begins with **Replacing** deficient levels of hormones and bringing you back to normalcy. When your testosterone levels are replenished, you restore vitality to each cell. It continues with **Repairing**. Once those hormones are in your system and operating properly, they will bring health on the cellular level, then to the organs of your body, and then to the various systems of your body. A replenished testosterone level is capable of defending against harmful elements, viruses and toxins. Then, the much-needed hormones **Restore** health and vitality to your entire body. When hormone levels are restored to optimal levels, health spreads! Finally, after only a few months on BHRT, you will feel **Revitalized**!

<u>Chapter 3 – Causes of Low Hormone Levels</u>

You might be asking, "What is causing my hormone levels to drop?"

There are a myriad of causes for declining hormone levels.

First, you have undoubtedly been exposed to **Phthalates**, which are a common type of environmental toxin.

There are phthalates in PVC piping, which is prevalent in most modern homes. "PVC" stands for "Poly Vinyl Chloride." When the PVC piping begins to break down, those foreign substances are released into the water supply and find their way into your body. This is the most dangerous endocrine disruptor there is, as it interferes with the actual formation of testosterone in your body. Think about that: all the water you drink and cook with in your home probably goes through that PVC piping, unless you have copper pipes.[ix]

This affects all of us, no matter what our age. For example, The World Health Organization (WHO) has seen testosterone levels in boys 6-12 years old decrease 24 - 34% in the last few years. The WHO calls this a "gender bender" that has caused obesity, Type 2 Diabetes, infertility, dementia, and loss of memory.[x] Thankfully, The WHO is currently campaigning to get PVC piping outlawed in our country.

Phthalates have been found in 100% of pregnant women, so this dangerous chemical is actually affecting babies in the womb. All of us suffer from these types of endocrine-disrupting chemicals. There is a specific signal that programs cells in your body to die. It's totally normal and healthy for 50 billion cells in your body to die every day! But studies have shown that phthalates can trigger what's known as "death-inducing signaling" in testicular cells, making them die earlier than they should.[xi] As a male, that scares me! Studies have linked phthalates to hormonal changes, lower sperm counts, less mobile sperm, birth defects in the male reproductive system, obesity, diabetes and thyroid irregularities.[xii]

Second, the population-wide decline in normal hormone levels may be the result of certain **Medications** we take.

For example, studies have shown that 35 - 50% of men will experience a decrease in their testosterone levels when on statins.[xiii] Statins are a class of lipid-lowering medications. They are typically prescribed for those who have heart disease and high cholesterol.

Third, your **Diet** and the foods you consume will affect your hormone levels.

High-grain diets are devastating. There is more "sugar content" in a bowl of oatmeal than in a root beer float and a bag of Twizzlers combined. Large amounts of sugar consumption cause Type 2 Diabetes. And those who suffer from that have a 57% decrease in their free testosterone levels.[xiv]

We all know consuming large amounts of sugar is not good for us. Eating too much sugar causes a barrage of symptoms including weight gain, abdominal obesity, decreased HDL and increased LDL, elevated triglycerides, high blood pressure, and increased uric acid levels.[xv]

The healthiest diets are paleo or ketogenic diets, which rely on healthy fats for energy, rather than glucose. Anytime you eat complex carbohydrates, like the kind found in grains, it turns into glucose, which is essentially, a form of sugar. It's better for your health if your body is a "fat-burning furnace" rather than a "glucose-burning furnace."

Fourth, **BPA Plastics** are dangerous and nearly everyone in this country faces exposure to them on a daily basis.

BPA stands for Bisphenol A. It is an industrial chemical that has been used to make certain plastics and resins since the 1960s. They are often used in containers that store food and beverages, such as water bottles. I would encourage you to use BPA-free products, to avoid microwaving plastics or putting them in the dishwasher, where the plastic may break down over time and allow BPA to leach into your foods.[xvi]

Fifth, **Lack of Sleep** can cause testosterone levels to plummet.

Our bodies were designed to get consistent, quality sleep. When you don't sleep well, it throws your body off. And one of the effects is a decrease in testosterone. When you are sleep-deficient, your body simply doesn't replenish testosterone naturally.[xvii] This can actually be a vicious cycle, because we need testosterone to enter REM cycles and sleep well, but low levels of testosterone can also cause lack of sleep. We lose both ways!

Sixth, and finally, various **Environmental Toxins** are dangerous.

Everything from air fresheners to perfumes to pesticides are potentially life-altering.

A study in England found the chemical **Atrazine** in abundance in lakes near certain pharmaceutical plants. Atrazine is an herbicide used by farmers to control destructive weeds. Researchers noticed there were no more male frogs in and around these lakes. They had all been converted to females during the embryo-genesis phase of their development. Now guess where much of that Atrazine ends up? In our corn, sorghum, sugar cane, and other foods.[xviii]

We are all being exposed to dangerous chemicals on a daily basis. Everyone is familiar with **Roundup,** the world's most widely used herbicide. Currently law suits are being filed against Roundup's maker, Monsanto, for a failure to warn farm workers and those in the forestry and landscaping industries of potential risks of cancer related to exposure to Roundup. But guess what? It's not just those farm workers who have been exposed. Studies have shown that 93% of us have traces of Roundup (Glyphosate) in our urine.[xix] And when those life-altering chemicals get into our bodies, they wreak havoc on our systems.

Chemicals such as **Aluminum** and **Mercury** are extremely dangerous to humans. Do you know the most common way those chemicals get into our bodies? It is not only through the environment, but through standard **Vaccines**. We are the most vaccinated country in the world, but despite all of our vaccines (or perhaps because of all of our vaccines), there are 33 other nations with lower infant mortality rates.[xx] We have the largest number of fetal deaths, and deaths in the first year of life of any wealthy, privileged Western nation. Stop and think about why that is, and what might be the cause of this extraordinarily tragic statistic. The Institute of Medicine (IOM) has finally admitted, "Vaccines are not free from side effects or adverse effects."[xxi]

Aluminum and mercury are endocrine-disrupting heavy metals that not only cause hormone imbalance, but create vitamin deficiencies within the body as well. Many of my patients have very low levels of Vitamin D. Recently, scholarly medical research papers were published linking "Low D" to "Low T." This new information was presented at The American Urological Association's 2015 Annual Meeting by Dr. Mary Ann McLaughlin, from the Mount Sinai Hospital in New York City.[xxii]

Exposure to **Fluoride** is a controversial topic, because fluoride is generally thought to be an essential component of dental hygiene and health. It is not only a common ingredient in toothpastes, mouthwashes, packaged teas and sodas, and pharmaceutical drugs, but many cities add fluoride to their water supply. Only sixteen countries in the world put fluoride in their water.[xxiii] The United States is one of them, and the results are shocking. Fluoride has been shown to weaken skeletal strength, cause arthritis, compromise the thyroid, calcify the pineal gland, accelerate female puberty, harm male and female fertility, negatively affect kidney health, harm the cardiovascular system, and have negative effects on the human brain and the ability to think clearly.[xxiv] The number one reason for poison control calls concerning fluoride are for children who have eaten toothpaste. Warning: Be aware of what is going into your body and the bodies of those you love!

Whether it is cosmetics you apply to your face, or synthetic sweeteners that have been added to your drinks and food, you are undoubtedly either ingesting or absorbing dangerous chemicals into your system that previous generations were never exposed to.

How to Protect Your Body Against Chemical Toxicity

The bottom line is this: you can still manage to live a healthy lifestyle, even in our modern world, which has become a minefield of toxins! Our bodies are unbelievable filters. We are designed to be able to battle all types of infections and diseases. We are designed to age gracefully and handle the challenges of growing older. That requires functioning optimally, so that we can thrive, not simply survive!

The engine oil and filter in your car were designed to lubricate and protect parts from contaminants and wear. But over time, those elements become thin and no longer protect the way they used to. Have you noticed how your car engine sounds different when you start it after you have run it 4,000 miles on the same oil? You can tell something is "not right." Only after you change the oil, will your car return to optimal performance. Changing your car's oil every 4,000-6,000 miles is crucial to its "health."

Your body functions the same way. Over time, hormone levels decrease. They must be renewed and restored. The pellet replacement therapy you will read about in this book starts with an initial insertion. Each pellet insertion lasts 4 to 6 months, until your body needs another "oil change." Coming into The Youth Institute and receiving a treatment will keep your hormone levels at their correct levels and your body functioning at its best.

Bio-identicals offer some measure of protection against the onslaught of environmental chemicals, food additives, preservatives, steroids, antibiotics and growth hormones found in our meat products, pesticides, herbicides, fungicides, and larvicides sprayed all over our vegetables, fluoride, chlorine, and pharmaceutical drugs in our water…. The list goes on and on.

You have the right to know that these things are harming you. And you should have the right to do something about it.

I believe in liberty and freedom. I believe in those principles with all my heart. I believe in our constitutional form of government that protects personal liberty. These are the rights that our forefathers intended. That includes being free as it relates to our health. We must be free to take our health matters into our own hands.

Chapter 4 – Consequences of Hormone Deficiency

When your hormone levels are low, that deficiency affects many parts of your body:

- You feel tired, drained, and "sapped" of energy

- You are susceptible to depression and despair

- You are at greater risk for heart attacks, blood clots and strokes

- You are more prone to diseases such as diabetes, dementia, and Alzheimer's

- You are more likely to get breast cancer, prostate cancer, and other types of cancer

- Your sex drive and sexual endurance will wane

What is Considered "Low?"

Today, testosterone levels for men are typically considered "normal" if they are anywhere from 301 to 1,197ng/dL. That's an absurdly vast range for what is accepted as normal! If I came to a sign in the road that signaled that there was a sharp curve ahead, but it said my acceptable speed could be anywhere from 20 mph to 70 mph, I'd see that as a very imprecise estimation of what my ideal speed should be to avoid losing control of my vehicle!

Where should my ideal hormone levels be as a man? Is 301 "normal" or is it a "new average" that I must be resigned to? I'll tell you. It's the new average. It's not where your grandfather and my grandfather were at ANY age. But because of all the things we've been discussing, it is now the new average. Here's the problem: the new average is not where your body needs to be! Big Pharma and the insurance companies have redefined what normal means. The "new normal," as insurance companies are calling it, is detrimental to the health of an entire generation of people. The numbers that are now regarded as commonplace are pitifully low in comparison to earlier generations, and our health as a society is suffering because of it. As of July 2017, lab standards have changed, referencing male levels of 264 - 916 ng/dL as "normal." Some universities have standards of 175 - 700 ng/dL as their reference range. Not only is this range far too wide, it is also far too low for optimal male health.

Using that average range for male testosterone, a study of 858 veterans over a 4.3-year period demonstrated that those in the bottom 25th percentile of testosterone levels had a 75% higher mortality rate.[xxv]

Another study by Dr. K.T. Khaw, published in 2007 in the online publication *Circulation*, proved that men with testosterone levels of 350 or lower, compared with men who had levels of 564 or higher, had a 41% higher mortality rate.[xxvi] **Clearly, the effects of low testosterone can be life-threatening**.

Our goal at The Youth Institute is to get your hormones back up to levels which are advantageous to your personal health, regardless of the fact that some conventional doctors might say that you are in a "normal range for your age." We are committed to finding your perfect hormonal balance, custom-tailored to your body, so you can have the energy, health and vitality that you desire.

The Effects of Low Testosterone

A study published by The National Institute of Health in 1990 found that half of healthy men between the ages of 50 and 70 years old have a testosterone level below the lowest levels seen in healthy men aged 20 to 40 years old.[xxvii] That means men are seeing a 50% decrease in their testosterone levels as they age into their 50s to 70s. Additional research goes back 60 years showing a trend of decreasing testosterone that continues to this day.

Dr. Molly M. Shores, writing in *The Archives of Internal Medicine* in 2006, described how a decrease in testosterone led to an 88% increase in mortality compared to men with higher testosterone levels.[xxviii]

Another study published by the National Institute of Health in 2002 revealed that when levels of testosterone are depleted, there is a much greater risk for arthrosclerosis.[xxix]

Dr. Abraham Morgentaler, the author of *Testosterone for Life*, describes many of the "soft symptoms" that are difficult to measure and even, at times, hard to describe. He calls it "The loss of one's Mojo."[xxx] I agree with him, because I've seen so many men come back to my office after receiving testosterone treatment. They are sleeping better, focusing better, having sex more often, and enjoying the energy and drive that they lacked before BHRT.

You only have one body.

You only have one life. How do you want to live it?

Chapter 5 – The Benefits of Hormone Replacement

So what happens when a person's hormone levels return to normal?

It is amazing, almost miraculous, to see the difference in your body when testosterone levels are abundant in the human body.

Research has shown that people with normal to high testosterone levels have:

~ Fewer heart attacks

~ Fewer blood clots

~ Fewer strokes

~ Reduced risk of diabetes

~ Reduced incidence of dementia

~ Reduced risk of Alzheimer's

~ Lower incidence of depression

~ Reduced risk of cancer

~ More energy

~ Greater sex drive

~ An ability to think clearly

In addition to the above list, many patients report reduced inflammation, reduced LDL (bad) cholesterol, improved mood, relief from dry eye syndrome, lower blood pressure, relief from the pain of arthritis, elimination of excess body fat, and the absence of chronic lumbar pain.

Look through that list. And ask yourself, "Who wouldn't want that?" I sure do. And those are the results I've seen in the lives of my patients at The Youth Institute for the last few years.

BHRT Protects Against Osteoporosis

One of the most widespread and crippling diseases is osteoporosis. Worldwide, osteoporosis causes more than 8.9 million fractures annually – that's an osteoporotic fracture every 3 seconds.[xxxi] Do we also want to call this a "new normal?" No! It might be a new average, but it is unacceptable.

Osteoporosis is estimated to affect 200 million women worldwide: 10% of women aged 60

20% of women aged 70

40% of women aged 80

66% of women aged 90[xxxii]

It affects an estimated 75 million people in Europe, USA and Japan.[xxxiii] During the year 2000, there were an estimated 9 million new osteoporotic fractures, of which 1.6 million were at the hip, 1.7 million were at the forearm, and 1.4 million were clinical vertebral fractures. Europe and the Americas accounted for 51% of all these fractures, while most of the remainder occurred in the Western Pacific region and Southeast Asia.[xxxiv] Worldwide, 1 in 3 women over age 50 will experience an osteoporotic fracture, as will 1 in 5 men over 50.[xxxv] Needless to say, it's a big problem.

So, what can we do? How can you take charge of your health to ensure you have the greatest chance of success in keeping your bone structure strong?

Hormone treatment has been proven to significantly increase bone density. But it matters what type of hormone treatment you use. The American Journal of Obstetrics and Gynecology has demonstrated the four-fold increase in bone density with bio-identical hormones over oral estrogen and a 2.5 times greater increase in bone density than with hormone patches. The details of those increases for women are:

~ 1-2% increase in bone density per year with oral estrogen

~ 3.5% increase in bone density per year with patches

~ 8.3% increase in bone density per year with pellet therapy[xxxvi]

In short, pellet BHRT has been shown to significantly increase bone density and to lessen the threat of osteoporosis.

This is just some of the evidence that is available in thousands of articles and studies published in medical journals. The weight of the evidence is overwhelming.

Again, I encourage you to do your own study and research. I believe you will come to the same strong conclusions I have about the effectiveness of hormone replacement therapy.

BHRT and Sexual Performance

Although the health benefits of hormone replacement are far-reaching, the benefit that is the most often asked about is the dramatic improvement of libido and sexual performance. Many of my patients, both men and women, are interested in enhancing the enjoyment of their sex lives. The changes are so profound that I have literally seen failing marriages saved because one or both partners started BHRT and suddenly had a renewed interest in a healthy, active sex life. It is well-documented that there is a direct correlation between normal to high hormone levels and increased libido, sexual interest, sexual performance, and sexual fulfillment. You can certainly expect to feel heightened sexual pleasure and interest if you begin bio-identical hormone replacement therapy as a primary benefit. Expect it to improve and strengthen your relationship with your life partner in a very powerful way!

Safety

What about the long-term implications of this treatment? "Cheerleaders" for synthetic hormone treatments sometimes assert that there are long-term dangers to bio-identicals, when, in fact, the reality is just the opposite. A collaborative analysis published in *The Journal of the National Cancer Institute* in 2008 found that there was no association between the risk of prostate cancer and any bio-identical hormone measured, including testosterone, DHT, estradiol, and others. This conclusion was reached after pooling the data from 18 separate studies that included 3,886 men with prostate cancer and 6,438 control subjects.[xxxvii] Sex hormones do not increase the risk of prostate cancer or any other kind of cancer!

Pellets Will Not Interact with Other Drugs

One of the clear advantages of using pellets as opposed to other forms of bio-identical replacement hormones is that there are no drug-to-drug interactions. Pellets are inserted into the fatty tissue of the hip and are absorbed over time directly into the bloodstream. They do not pass through the digestive system like most prescription drugs, and they are not metabolized by the liver. This is an extremely safe method of delivery and most closely mimics your own body's natural process of secreting hormones. For this reason, pellets are ideal for people on oral medications or for people with clotting disorders.

Supportive Medical Literature

I have on my computer and in my office, thousands of articles on hormone therapy and its benefits. Because of the small size and streamlined nature of this book, I can only mention a few of those articles here. In the future, I am planning to write a longer, medically-oriented book for those who wish to learn about this subject in-depth. However, until that time, we have many of these articles available for your perusal, both on our website and in our office. I wholeheartedly encourage you to study, to do your own research, and to investigate what modern, progressive doctors and researchers are finding.

These documented studies show the positive effects of hormone treatment on our cardiovascular systems, our nervous systems, and our metabolic systems. They demonstrate how the overall effects of aging can prevent your body from performing optimally. And they prove that BHRT is a kind of "age reversal" therapy that has numerous positive effects on our health and sexual performance.

When your body is optimally balanced, you will not be as susceptible to disease. As I have said earlier, nothing is a panacea. But we all want our bodies to be functioning as efficiently as possible, as they were designed to.

The following are the most compelling reasons to begin bio-identical hormone replacement therapy:

1. There is an abundance of evidence that replacing lost hormones is essential to good health.

2. Replacing low and declining hormones is best done with bio-identical hormones. This is the only kind of hormone that is equal to what your body naturally produces and therefore, is completely safe, without any of the negative side effects.

I will continue discussing the last point in the next chapter...

Chapter 6 – What are Bio-identical Hormones?

Bio-identical hormones are the safest and most natural form of hormone replacement available, because they are created using familiar, plant-based ingredients like yams, soy, or olive oil. The Mayo Clinic has defined bio-identical hormones as "compounds that have exactly the same chemical and molecular structure as hormones that are produced in the human body." [xxxviii] This means that the body recognizes bio-identical hormones as its own. This is critical. Conventional hormone replacement therapy uses drugs that are dangerous chemical compounds. Their structure is likely to have adverse consequences on the human organism.

Hormones are not drugs. Hormones are special regulatory substances that are created in the endocrine glands and transported in the blood to stimulate specific tissues into action. They are made up of signaling molecules that target organs to regulate physiology and behavior. Bio-identicals do not come with the undesirable side effects of traditional hormone drugs because they are identical, chemically speaking, to those made by your own body. [xxxix]

Bio-identical hormones are infinitely safer, because they are the structural duplicates to the hormones your body made a lot of when you were young. *Hence, the term "bio-identical," as in, "identical to your own biology."*

The Youth Institute Pellet

The pellets that we use at The Youth Institute are made up of 99.5% natural testosterone that comes from yams. Their chemical structure is **molecularly identical** to the testosterone made in your own body. The other 0.5% of the pellet is composed of steric acid which allows the testosterone to hold together and to dissolve slowly after placement. This "**identical-ness"** is the **major differentiator** between bio-identical and synthetic hormones. Your body will not reject or react against bio-identicals. Unlike synthetic hormones that have dangerous side effects, BHRT is safe and effective.

The History of Pellets

The testosterone hormone was first isolated by researchers in the early 1930s. The very first scholarly paper published on testosterone pellet therapy was in a British Journal in 1935. Pellet Therapy was then approved for medical use in 1939. That's nearly 80 years ago! BHRT is not something new. It has been around a long time and its safety has been proven for far longer than the majority of prescription drugs so many Americans are taking.

Why We Use Pellets

There are several different methods of delivery of bio-identical hormones, including creams, gels, troches, pills, injections, and pellets. All of the above are better than taking synthetic hormones! However, the best and most effective method of bio-identical hormone delivery is the insertion of pellets, and that is why we use pellets exclusively at The Youth Institute.

Bio-identical pellet treatments mimic your ovary and testicle production identically. When a topical cream is used instead, the testosterone is not absorbed as readily through the skin and the results are limited. Similarly, when pills are taken orally, not enough of the hormone is absorbed through the digestive tract. And treatment through intravenous injections are outlawed for women. They are available for men only, and even with that method, testosterone injections result in levels that mimic a roller coaster, with up-and-down surges of high and low hormone levels.

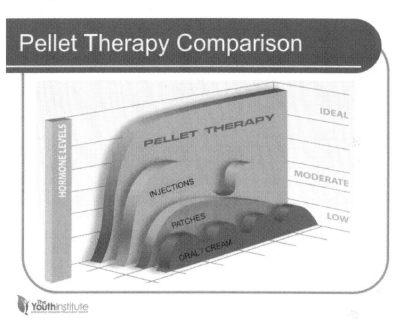

Pellet therapy is the only method of treatment that allows your hormone levels to remain constant for months at a time, exactly the way your body does naturally, producing a steady supply of hormones that flow directly into the bloodstream. As you work out, your blood flow increases, and more testosterone flows through your system, just as it was designed to do. Pellet therapy is ideal, because it provides a steady supply of life-giving hormones. The pellets also act as a "reservoir." When the heart rate increases, more testosterone is transported into the bloodstream.

Since the pellet dissolves over time, you will want to get "placed" again after about 4 months. Why so soon, if the pellet is designed to last up to 6 months? Because you never want to go too low ever again. Getting "placed" again after 4 months will prevent you from "bottoming out," sending your body into a downward spiral of feeling lethargic, mentally unfocused and devoid of a healthy libido.

The Benefits of Our Pellet Therapy

Take a moment and read through the benefits of *BHRT* listed below. Does this sound like the positive health model you have been looking for?

The Benefits of Bio-Identical Hormones	
Safe	Lowers your risk of depression
Absorbed directly into the blood	Lowers your risk of cancer
Lowers your chance of diabetes	Increases your energy level
Lowers cholesterol	Creates a strong sex drive
Lowers your chance of obesity	Lowers your risk of heart attacks
Improves clarity	Lowers your risk for blood clots
Improves cognitive ability	Lowers your risk of a stroke
Lowers your risk of Alzheimer's	Lowers your risk of dementia
Increases lean muscle mass	Increases bone density

In fact, the dangers of bio-identical hormones are so minimal, I would venture to say that it is more dangerous *not to be on them*. That is the degree of protection they offer against various types of ailments as we get older. There are, of course, a few minor side effects, which I will discuss in a later chapter. They are however, truly minor in comparison to the extraordinary benefits of BHRT.

It is the conclusion of doctors and researchers all around the world that bio-identical hormone replacement therapy is safe, proven, and effective.

Safe

I have read extensively about the safety of BHRT and I have never seen any research that revealed any significant health risks. The research shows there are no major dangers associated with this treatment.

Proven

Through our website, you will have access to thousands of scientific articles that outline the proven results of BHRT.

Effective

I've seen the phenomenal changes in thousands of lives at The Youth Institute in the last 7 years.

"Safe, proven, and effective" are the words I would use to describe bio-identical hormones! In the next chapter, we will look at two vastly different methods of treatment that are available today: synthetic hormone replacement vs. bio-identical hormone replacement. And we will see that BHRT is the safest and most effective hormone therapy available.

Chapter 7 – <u>The Difference Between Bio-identical Hormones and Synthetic Hormones</u>

Why is there so much controversy surrounding hormones?

It is important to understand that The Center for Disease Control (CDC) and The Federal Drug Administration (FDA) group all types of hormones together. According to their classifications, there is no difference between synthetic and bio-identical hormones. They lump them together in the same category, and assume that because synthetic hormones are dangerous, bio-identicals must be dangerous as well.

This is a false assumption.

There is a world of difference between the two.

For example, governmental regulatory agencies classify both natural progesterone and medroxyprogesterone (or MPA) as progestins. But these two progestins are very different. They may produce some of the same effects in the body, but they are vastly different in terms of their chemical makeup, how they are manufactured, what sources they are derived from, and how the body ultimately responds to them long-term.

In fact, the disparity between these two products is so significant, it can be a matter of life and death. Studies have shown that natural progesterone actually *decreases* the likelihood of breast cancer, while synthetic progesterone (MPA), *increases* its likelihood by up to 69%.

So, you see, "progestin" is a very broad classification. To discover whether a progestin is dangerous or safe, we must look at the source and structure of that hormone.

If the ingredients sourced to create a hormone are foreign to the human body, it is far more likely to pose dangers and harmful repercussions.

If the ingredients are sourced from food, and are identical to those produced naturally in the human body, it makes sense that the body would receive them positively.

All the research on this subject makes clear and evident the fact that the complications and problems associated with hormone replacement are found only when using synthetics, both because of their chemical makeup and their mode of application. The synthetic progestins, such as MPA, undeniably increase the likelihood of breast cancer. [xl]

Bio-identicals, on the other hand, and in particular, pellet therapy, mimic the body's natural process, with the gradual release of an organic substance over a period of several months. I have administered bio-identicals to thousands of my patients with great success and have found no major negative side effects.

The bottom line? We should put only what is natural to our bodies inside of our bodies.

Drug Companies are Intentionally Creating Confusion

I had a patient ask me the other day, "Why is it that, all of a sudden, I am seeing ads everywhere on television, in drug stores, and in magazines, advertising hormone replacement therapy and testosterone boosters?

Those advertisements and therapies weren't around when I was a kid. Why now? Was it just me not noticing them, or is this truly a new problem or even a fad? And the lingo is confusing. Not only do I hear about 'hormone replacement therapy,' but now I'm seeing ads for 'bio-equivalent hormones.' What's this? Is it the same thing? I'm confused. What's the difference?"

Those are good questions - questions that I have been asked by thousands of clients I've treated successfully. With a background in obstetrics and gynecology, I want both women and men to experience health and vigor, and to age gracefully.

As I said earlier in the book, after years of being uninformed about these topics, I began investigating with an open mind. I discovered how, with the right hormone treatment, we can achieve that younger, stronger, more energetic, and sexier reality. But it must be the right treatment … with the right hormones.

When it comes to replenishing hormone levels in our bodies, we have two options to choose from: synthetic hormone replacement or bio-identical hormone replacement. Let's look more closely at the differences between these two methods of treatment, the benefits and dangers of each, and come to a rational conclusion about which is best for both men and women today.

First, if a substance is introduced into your body, and your body cannot metabolize it or break it down, that causes problems. Synthetic hormones, as we will see, are made from substances that are foreign to our systems.

Second, the television ads touting synthetic hormones refer to them as "bio-equivalent." This term has been coined precisely because it sounds so similar to the term "bio-identical." The pharmaceutical companies selling synthetic hormones want you to believe that "bio-equivalent" and "bio-identical" are the same. They are deliberately creating confusion around these two terms. But the differences between these two products are vast.

Our consumerist marketplace is rife with clever marketing tactics designed to reassure an unsuspecting buyer. For example, because of the dramatic increase in the consumption of organic foods, many food manufacturers have started labeling their products as "natural," hoping that most consumers will equate the term "organic" with "natural." Many people assume that natural food is safe, minimally processed, hormone-free, antibiotic-free and chemical-free. The reality is, neither the FDA nor the USDA has any rules or regulations in place for companies to claim that their products are natural – only a loose set of guidelines that are not enforced. Ultimately, any food manufacturer is free to use this term on its food packaging, regardless of the ingredients it contains.

"Organic" foods however, are regulated by extremely strict guidelines. They must contain no synthetic pesticides, herbicides, fertilizers, antibiotics or growth hormones. Organic farmers are subject to frequent unannounced certification inspections by third-party inspectors. Organic growers and food producers go through extremely rigorous testing for the privilege of placing the term "organic" on their packaging.[xli] As a result, the quality of a product that is labeled "organic" is usually far superior to one labeled "natural," even though those two terms might appear to be indistinguishable at first glance.

This comparison illustrates why it's important to be educated and aware of who wants to sell you what! The pharmaceutical industry wants you to think "bio-equivalent" and "bio-identical" are the same, exactly the way industrial food producers want you to think "organic" and "natural" are the same thing. Pay close attention to the phraseology of the companies trying to get you to spend your money on their products!

Synthetic Hormone Replacement Therapy

For years, doctors have prescribed synthetic hormone treatment for women who were menopausal. The two most common hormones prescribed are Premarin and Provera. With the best of intentions, doctors gave these drugs to women who were experiencing menopausal symptoms such as hot flashes, night sweats, hair loss, poor sleep, anxiety, and depression.

It is important to realize that Premarin and Provera are not natural. They are chemical compounds that are alien to the human body. And they cause some very dangerous side effects.

Premarin is a conjugated equine estrogen (CEE) that is derived from the urine of a pregnant horse. Women, do you really want something made from horse urine in your body? Think about that for a moment. Does it make sense to introduce a chemical long-term that is completely unfamiliar to your genetic make-up? Premarin changes the normal ratio of Estradiol to Estrone (two forms of estrogen) in a woman's body from 2:1 to 1:2. This in and of itself is unnatural.

Provera is another synthetic chemical made from medroxyprogesterone acetate, which is a chemical derivative of progesterone, however, it offers none of the positive benefits of natural progesterone. A high percentage of women who start taking

Provera discover that the side effects are so uncomfortable that they discontinue its use.

Dangers Associated with Synthetic Hormones

Some of the dangers and common side effects of **Premarin** include: increased risk of breast cancer, blood clots, high blood pressure, fluid retention, headaches, leg cramps, increased risk of stroke, gall stones, tenderness of the breasts, worsened uterine fibroids, increased risk of diabetes, worsened endometriosis, increased risk of endometrial cancer, impaired glucose tolerance, nausea and vomiting.[xlii]

Similarly, some of the possible side effects of taking **Provera** are: hair loss or hair growth, depression, fluid retention, skin rashes, breast tenderness, weight gain, acne, impaired glucose tolerance, menstrual irregularities, blood clots, breast cancer and birth defects.[xliii]

Prempro, a pill combining both Premarin and Provera, has been shown to cause an increase in breast cancer by 26% after 4 years of ingestion.

The Women's Health Initiative (WHI) was a long-term national health study focused on strategies for preventing heart disease, breast and colorectal cancer, and osteoporotic fractures in postmenopausal women. In 2002, WHI proved that synthetic hormones cause breast cancer, heart attacks, strokes, dementia, and blood clots.[xliv]

In 2004, the results of The Women's Health Initiative Memory Study were released. Their research proved conclusively that not only was Prempro failing to protect women from declining mental capacity, it actually doubled the risk of dementia for women who took the drug.[xlv]

Bio-identicals vs. Synthetics

An article was published in the 2005 issue of The Journal of Cancer regarding a study that analyzed the health of over 54,000 female patients. Half of the patients were treated with a combination of bio-identical estrogen and bio-identical progesterone. The other half were treated with a combination of bio-identical estrogen and synthetic progesterone. The first group had a 10% decrease in the incidence of breast cancer. The group that was treated with the synthetic progesterone saw an increase in the incidence of breast cancer by 40%.[xlvi]

Two years later, a follow-up study analyzed the health of another 80,000 women over a longer period of time. **The researchers reported zero cases of breast cancer in the bio-identical group and a 69% increase of cases of breast cancer in the synthetic progesterone group.**[xlvii]

Here's my question: Why would you want to ingest any foreign substance such as horse urine, when there are better, more effective, and healthier alternatives? Why would you want to do that to yourself?

If you are a horse suffering from hormone imbalance, then Premarin might be just what you need! But if you aren't, I strongly encourage you to stay away from it, or any of its derivatives.

My Patient, Jan

Jan, one of my OB/GYN patients came to see me in my office recently, dissatisfied with the Premarin she was on, and scared of the side effects she was reading about. Her initial reaction was to get off hormones completely, but she knew what the consequences were of discontinuing hormone therapy entirely.

We talked for a while, and as I described the alternative of bio-identical hormone treatment, she lit up with excitement. Was it possible that there could be a solution that was both safe and effective?

Within 2 months of starting treatment, Jan returned to see me, elated with the results and relieved of her fears. She said, "I feel like I have my life back again." She did, and without the dangerous side effects of synthetic treatment.

My Experience Prescribing Both Types of Hormones

As an OB/GYN, when I prescribed Premarin, I never got the opportunity to follow up with a patient and monitor her blood labs. I just prescribed the drug. Besides which, the conventional drugs used to treat menopause such as Premarin and Estrace do nothing to lower a woman's FSH level, which is really what she needs to relieve her symptoms.

I have a unique background, being a doctor who has treated thousands of menopausal women, both with conventional drugs, and with bio-identical hormones. There are very few doctors out there who have had the experience of treating so many women and observing the effects of both forms of hormone treatment on their patients. I can tell you beyond a shadow of a doubt, after having plenty of exposure to and familiarity with both, that bio-identicals are by far and away the superior method of treatment in terms of safety and effectiveness.

Synthetic Hormones are Unnatural

To summarize, here is my case against the use of synthetic hormones in replacement therapy:

• Synthetic hormones are unnatural and foreign to the human body. Premarin is made from a pregnant horse's urine and contains more potent estrogens than the human body can handle.

• The body has serious trouble assimilating synthetic hormones and, in fact, will react against them. Conjugated estrogens are estrogen products that contain blended equine estrogens including estrone sulfate, equilin sulfate, and equilenin sulfate. Taken orally, they must pass through the liver before entering the blood system, and that is where the problems occur. Estrogens are primarily metabolized by the liver, and conjugated estrogens inhibit the production of bile, sometimes causing jaundice. Premarin has also been known to elevate liver enzymes, causing a rise in clotting factors, which increases the chances of clots in the veins and lungs.

When bio-identical pellets are the method of hormone replacement therapy used, there is no danger to the liver. Pellets are inserted into the fatty tissue of the buttocks, and dissolve there over time. Hormones will be absorbed naturally and gradually into the bloodstream without ever even passing through the liver. In addition, bio-identical hormones are not nearly as potent as those conjugated estrogens from horses.

• The side effects of Premarin, Provera, Prempro, and other conjugated estrogen products are dangerous and well-documented. Simply put, they cause more problems than they solve.

• Synthetic hormones are formulated to treat symptoms, but do not get to the root of the problem.

Chapter 8 – Hormone Replacement for Women

Let me put my OB/GYN hat on and talk first to the women, specifically about changes in their levels of testosterone, estrogen, and progesterone.

Changes in Testosterone

Women need testosterone. It's not just a "man's hormone!" In the past, testosterone levels in an average 20-year old woman might have been between 70 - 90 ng/dL. What I am seeing in today's women are ranges much lower: between 8 - 30 ng/dl. By the time those women reach the age of 50, their levels will drop even more significantly - to between 2 - 10 ng/dL. (This measurement is an abbreviation for "Nanograms Per Decilitre." A decilitre measures fluid volume that is 1/10 of a litre.) On the average, women are losing 3% of their testosterone each year. By menopause, women have lost 70-90% of their total testosterone.

At The Youth Institute, we restore a woman's testosterone level to somewhere between 90 – 200 ng/dl. Female T levels are not considered high unless they are over 200. I routinely find the most advantageous T level for each one of my female patients. The higher her T level, the greater her libido and energy level, however, we don't want to go so high that she starts to see side effects, such as clitoromegaly, an enlargement of the clitoris. This is a careful balancing act with each female patient.

In 1996, a clinical study was conducted by treating Alzheimer's patients with testosterone. Although there is no cure for Alzheimer's, the researchers proved that the disease could be slowed. Their patients experienced some regression and some very positive outcomes. [xlviii] Other similar studies confirm the therapeutic effects of testosterone on the human brain. [xlix]

Women benefit from healthy levels of testosterone!

The human body is like a finely tuned engine. It converts cholesterol into hormones that are necessary for optimal functioning. The diagram below illustrates the conversion of cholesterol to progesterone, testosterone and estrogen.

Method of Enzymatic Breakdown of Testosterone (*Diagram*):

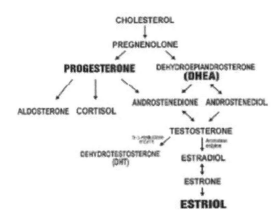

Changes in Estrogen

Estrogen is produced during the menstrual cycle by a maturing ovum. When the estrogen in a woman's body reaches 200pg/ml, that triggers her anterior pituitary to release luteinizing hormone, which causes ovulation. Menstruating women produce estrogen from the time their periods start as teenagers, until menopause. Levels can fluctuate from 50 to 400 pg/ml throughout their cycles.

At menopause, a woman's body stops producing estrogen and over time, her levels of estrogen drop to zero.

This may lead to a variety of symptoms, including:

~ PMS, irregular menstrual cycles, heavy bleeding

~ weight gain

~ decreased sex drive, mood swings, depression

~ thyroid dysfunction

~ fibroids, endometriosis

~ gallbladder problems

~ breast tenderness, fibrocystic breasts

Changes in Progesterone

Progesterone, testosterone and estradiol are all made in the ovaries. The corpus luteum in the ovaries is the primary site of progesterone production in women, although progesterone is also produced in smaller quantities by the adrenal glands. If a woman becomes pregnant, her progesterone levels will continue to rise. Progesterone prepares the lining of the uterus to except a fertilized egg. During a woman's monthly cycle, progesterone peaks after ovulation, a time when most women seem to feel their best.

Levels of progesterone begin to decline, commonly by age 35. At this time, women may notice changes in their periods, such as prolonged bleeding and/or shorter times between menstrual cycles. They may also experience mood swings and have more trouble sleeping. It is at this point that many women complain to their doctors about anxiety, sleeping problems, and depression. That is why progesterone can be thought of as the anti-stress hormone.

In addition to receiving estrogen and testosterone in the form of bio-identical pellets, women who still have an intact uterus would also be prescribed progesterone at our clinic. For women who have had a hysterectomy, the progesterone would be optional. The reason being, studies have shown that estrogen therapy without progesterone therapy can increase the chances of endometrial cancer, therefore the addition of natural progesterone eliminates this concern for women who still have an intact uterus.

However, taking progesterone has many irrefutable benefits even if a woman no longer has a uterus, including blood sugar regulation, the promotion of normal sleep patterns, and the stimulation of new bone. So women who have undergone a hysterectomy may choose to take progesterone anyway.

Women have the option of taking natural progesterone using one of the following delivery methods:

1. It can be absorbed transdermally with a cream that is rubbed into the skin at night.

2. It can be prescribed in the form of a "troche" which is a small medicated lozenge designed to dissolve on the tongue.

3. Prometrium is a patented form of bio-identical progesterone that comes in a pill form in 100 and 200 mg. doses and is taken orally in the evening.

All three forms of progesterone are made from plant sources like yams, olive oil, and soy, and will protect the uterus from cancer. They are all useful as a treatment for the symptoms of perimenopause and menopause.

A Normal Menstrual Cycle

In the chart below, you will see graphed changes in the levels of estrogen and progesterone throughout a women's menstrual cycle.

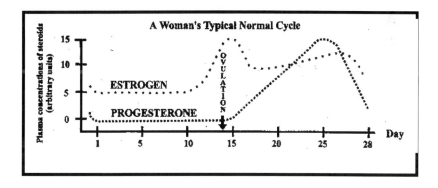

But where are the testosterone levels in this diagram? Graphically speaking, they would be way at the top of the page. What is the reason for this? Remember this equation:

T = 10 x E

In other words, T is the Testosterone Level and E is the Estrogen Level. Your testosterone level should, ideally, be ten times your estrogen level. However, a normal woman's menstrual cycle affects her hormone levels, and so her levels fluctuate up and down more than a man's throughout any given month.

Women, the important aspects to note here are:

~ The menstrual cycle occurs in two phases. The beginning of the cycle is known as the follicular phase and the final part of the cycle is considered the luteal phase. Midway through the cycle, between days 12 and 16, is when ovulation occurs.

~ The levels of estrogen and progesterone fluctuate consistently through every menstrual cycle.

~ When you know how a normal menstrual cycle works, you are able to understand the symptoms of premenstrual syndrome (PMS), perimenopause, and menopause. These symptoms are often the result of hormone imbalance.

~ An irregular menstrual cycle is a good indicator of hormonal imbalance.

Symptoms of Menopause

When a woman's hormone levels drop, she will begin to enter into menopause, where common symptoms include:

~ Menstrual periods that occur less frequently and eventually cease

~ Heart pounding or racing

~ Hot flashes (usually worst during the first 1 or 2 years)

~ Night sweats

~ Skin flushing

~ Problems sleeping

~ Decreased interest in sex or changes in sexual response

~ Forgetfulness

~ Headaches

~ Mood swings including irritability and anxiety

~ Urine leakage

~ Vaginal dryness and painful sexual intercourse

~ Vaginal infections

~ Joint aches and pains

Can you relate to some or all of these?

Lab tests can be performed to look for changes in hormone levels. Test results can help determine if you are close to or have already gone through menopause. Lab tests may include Estradiol, Follicle-stimulating hormone (FSH), and Luteinizing hormone (LH), Testosterone, Free Testosterone, Thyroid Panel w/Thyroid Stimulating Hormone, T3 Uptake, Total T4 , Free T4 Index, Progesterone, Complete Blood Count and Vitamin D.

BHRT is the "Cure" for Menopause

Women, the most important thing to remember is that you don't need to fear "the change of life." If you are approaching perimenopause, you are in the throes of menopause, or menopause has already come and gone, BHRT can alleviate any symptoms you may have. In fact, BHRT prevents you from going through dramatic symptoms associated with "the change" for as long as you are on it. You will most likely, continue to ovulate as long as your ovaries are intact and functional. This is healthy for your body and will preserve your health and your looks for a much longer time.

One patient asked me, "So, will I be able to get pregnant when I'm 75?" The answer to that is no. At a certain point, your ovaries will stop releasing eggs. You will certainly continue to ovulate for longer than you might have without the bio-identicals, but even on hormone replacement therapy, your ovaries will cease to be functional as you reach your mature years.

After starting bio-identicals, if a woman's uterus is still intact, but she has gone through menopause, she will be given both estrogen and progesterone to avoid resuming her menstrual cycle, which is undesirable to most women. The majority of the time, women will not have a full-on period, but they may have some break-through bleeding. The relief of other post-menopausal symptoms is so great that usually the minimal amount of bleeding from time to time is simply a minor inconvenience.

If and when breakthrough bleeding first occurs, we ask that our female patients see their regular gynecologists to have it evaluated. Reason being, sometimes bleeding can be an indication of another problem unrelated to hormone therapy, such as polyps, fibroids, or endometrial cancer. In the vast majority of cases, our patients' work-ups will prove to be benign. The spotting is usually just the result of restoring the sex hormones to youthful levels. (Imagine your uterus is asleep, and I'm going to wake it up!) However, if spotting does occur, a thorough evaluation by a gynecologist is a precautionary measure that ultimately protects you from overlooking a more serious issue.

Ladies, I will be happy to talk with you about your personal situation during our one-on-one consultation and answer any questions you may have regarding BHRT and how it can prevent the symptoms of menopause forever.

Who Can Benefit from BHRT?

First and foremost, women suffering from the symptoms of perimenopause or menopause (listed above) will experience immediate and life-long relief. It is also particularly restorative for women who have had a full or partial hysterectomy.

In addition, bio-identicals can treat and improve a wide spectrum of other problems, including: Chronic Fatigue Syndrome, Post Traumatic Stress Disorder, depression, autoimmune diseases, hypothyroidism, metabolic syndrome, weight gain, low energy, insomnia, osteoporosis, low libido, adrenal fatigue, PMS, memory loss, and migraines.

<u>Chapter 9 – Hormone Replacement for Men</u>

Now, let me speak to the men.

As a man ages, his hormone levels drop as well. Optimal testosterone levels for a man are between 800 and 1,200 ng/dL. But I see men come into my office every day with levels in the 100s and 200s.

You will notice on the chart below that today, men's testosterone levels typically decrease as they age.

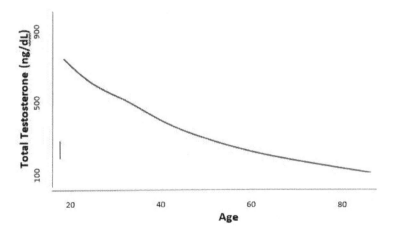

This graph should alert us to the changes that are happening in our bodies. Something is different. And that difference has dramatic effects.

Think of your body as an engine. In your twenties, that engine was firing away on all 8 cylinders. You had energy, focus, concentration, sexual drive, muscle mass and a great memory. You were a warrior!

But something started happening in your mid-thirties. At first, the change was almost imperceptible. Soon, you began noticing that you could not do the things you used to. You became irritable and anxious.

Things were "different" sexually. That once-powerful 8-cylinder engine was now down to 3 or 4 cylinders, and you could feel the effects.

These "engine problems" are something previous generations did not experience, at least not to the degree we are seeing today. Men's testosterone levels have been steadily declining since the 1960s. In 2007, an article published in The Journal of Clinical Endocrinology and Metabolism reported that the average American man is experiencing a sinking testosterone level that goes down about 1% per year. In other words, 50-year old men today have, on average, testosterone levels that are 38% lower than 50-year old men from 1980.[i] A similar study in Denmark revealed that testosterone levels have been declining for decades in other parts of the world as well.[li]

The Effects of Low Testosterone in Men

There are many signs and symptoms of testosterone deficiency in men as they age. They may experience one or more of the following symptoms:

~ Anxiety

~ Irritability

~ Fatigue

~ Loss of energy

~ Poor focus

~ Poor concentration

~ Depression

~ Osteoporosis

~ Decrease in sexual interest

~ Restless leg syndrome

~ Higher LDL cholesterol

~ Arthritis

~ Alzheimer's

~ Weight gain (despite exercising)

~ Loss of memory

~ A general loss of muscle mass and tone

~ Decreased nocturnal erections

~ Inability to maintain a hard erection

~ Heart attack

~ Stroke

~ Diabetes

~ Hypertension

~ Loss of confidence

Is any of that "normal?" No. *It might be common, but it is not normal.* Something is wrong ... and we know it. It is not the way God designed our bodies to age. We are meant to live full, passionate and active lives throughout our 40s, 50s, 60s, 70s and 80s.

It's No Longer Just an "Aging" Issue

Unfortunately, there is more to this sad story. I am seeing something at The Youth Institute that I never thought I would see. Young men in their late teens and twenties come into my office with testosterone levels dangerously low - in the 100s and sometimes below that. Some of these men are returning from serving our country in military service in Afghanistan and Iraq. Others are in college or just starting their careers. They are depressed, lethargic, and sometimes suicidal. They have lost sexual interest and have changed from the warriors they once were to being complacent couch potatoes.

However, the beauty of bio-identical hormone replacement therapy is that is effective, regardless of age and no matter what the cause of low testosterone can be linked to.

Men, the good news is, you don't need to dread getting older anymore! You can still be the warriors you were created to be ... long into your 70s and 80s.

Natural testosterone not only helps a 50 year-old man feel like he is 30 again, it protects his overall health.

Chapter 10 – Becoming a Patient at The Youth Institute

By now, you might be wondering, "How do I get started? What's the process of becoming a patient at The Youth Institute?"

The Initial Consultation

Your first step is to call one of our 4 clinics and set up a consultation appointment. We'll sit down and talk one-on-one in the privacy of my office. Feel free to take as much time as you need to address your concerns. I look forward to meeting you!

Recently, a new patient named Sally came into my office. She had a lot of questions. I mean, A LOT of questions. She had talked with her personal physician, she had read articles, and she had talked with friends. All that added up to about 40 questions she had written down on a legal pad.

We went through them one by one. Several times I pointed her to additional articles that are available on our website. By the end of our visit, I had answered all of her questions. But she still needed some time to decide if BHRT was right for her. I understood her need to take things slowly and make an informed decision.

I told her, "It's your body. It's your decision. No one can or should make that decision for you."

Sally called back 2 days later. We scheduled her for labs, and 2 days after that, she was back in our office receiving her first pellet placement. If you talked with her today, she would tell you, "That was the best decision I ever made." But it was made only after careful investigation and reflection.

I also frequently hold public seminars, which are another great opportunity to get all your questions answered, and listen to the concerns of other prospective patients like you.

Labs

After our consultation, the next step is putting in an order for your lab work. You can choose to have your blood drawn that day if you like, or whenever it's convenient. The lab tests are very easy and quick. It's a simple blood draw that can be done at any local blood lab such as Labcorp. I will send the necessary order for the tests to be done, called a "blood lab requisition" to the lab of your choice. You can visit the lab on your own schedule. It usually takes 5 to 15 minutes, depending on the schedule of the lab. I receive the results back on my desk within 12 to 24 hours.

In our Cary office, we have a phlebotomist on staff, so the turnaround for labs there is even more expeditious.

Pellet Placement

Once I receive your labs, our administrative assistant will call you to schedule an appointment for your first pellet placement. Using your lab results, I will personalize a BHRT pellet treatment specifically for you. When you come back into our office, it takes no more than 10 to 15 minutes for the placement procedure. I will re-consult with you, with your lab results in hand, and then do the quick and easy placement, which is an outpatient procedure performed in our clinic. After a pellet placement, you may return to work or normal daily activities, but it is recommended that you take it easy for the rest of the day. No vigorous exercise!

At that time, our office staff will give you specific instructions for caring for the bandage and tape that protect the incision area. A member of our friendly staff will call you the next day to make sure you are doing well and to answer any other questions you may have at that time. It is very simple to get started and you'll be feeling the effects of the pellets in no time!

The Dosing Model

The dosing model is crucial to the overall success of this program for all my patients. After doing this for many years, administering thousands of placements, I utilize an algorithm that indicates what is best for each individual patient according to his/her labs. The algorithms are derived from information based on thousands of patients, which makes me extremely confident in my ability to design a treatment plan that will work perfectly for you.

I hope you see immediate results and a positive impact on your health and vitality in the short term. However, I chose BHRT for the long-term results; to prevent things like arthrosclerosis, dementia, and diabetes, which is just as important, if not more so. It's similar to taking vitamins every day. I may or may not feel the short-term benefits of daily supplementation, but I know I am building a strong foundation for long-term health. Similarly, we jog, work out, and eat the right foods so that we're healthy now, and will be healthy in the future.

Dosage for Females

Regarding pre-menopausal women, I am especially concerned with their testosterone levels. We will get them checked with the labs and make sure they are high enough. A staff member from The Youth Institute will call you the next day to see how you are doing, and we will also re-check the labs in 4 to 6 weeks. We'll monitor how you feel and continue to analyze your blood work over time.

In general, I like to make sure that my female patients maintain a testosterone level of between 90 – 200 ng/dl. Appropriate levels for a woman's progesterone and estrogen will vary based on her time of life, and we can discuss what is optimal for you when we meet.

Dosage for Men

At The Youth Institute, when we run labs for our male patients, we pay especially close attention to their testosterone level, which, ideally, should be over 800 ng/dl.

Too often, I am seeing men (even men in their 20s) who have such low testosterone (oftentimes in the 100s, or lower!) that it really concerns me. I will run their levels through our Youth Institute algorithm and come up with a dosage plan that includes the number of pellets they will receive. Once treated, we check back in 4 to 6 weeks with new lab tests, and invariably, our patients' levels rise dramatically.

I want to find out who you are and what's best for you. That's why the subjective part of my record-keeping is so important.

Subjective and Objective Data

At The Youth Institute, the careful monitoring of each patient is based on both objective and subjective data. Subjective data is information from the patient's point of view, including symptoms, feelings, and experiences reported first-hand from those receiving BHRT.

Objective data is observable and/or measurable data from the physician's point of view, obtained through observation, physical examination, and laboratory testing. I believe it is important to pay close attention to both to achieve the best results for all of my patients.

Why is the subjective data so important? Because the most significant determining factor in whether or not BHRT is working should be how the patient feels. Although the labs are important, how YOU FEEL is the reason for the therapy. The external, objective data will simply confirm what you are telling me.

Ongoing Consultations

After your initial consultation with me, I will never charge you again for another consultation. What happens if you have questions the next week or the next month? Schedule an appointment. Come on in. I am here for you anytime you need a question answered. I encourage all my patients to do additional research. Bring articles to me that you've read. I want you to know more than I know. It's your body. Take charge of it.

Patient History

It is very important that I receive a complete and accurate picture of your health history before we begin treatment. This includes all current medications you take, and vitamin supplements. Any illnesses you suffer from should be fully disclosed, such as diabetes, hypertension, liver, kidney or heart disease, a history of stroke or cancer, HIV, or clotting disorders. You should also be under the care and supervision of a general physician and receive standard yearly examinations. You must be at least 18 years of age to receive pellet therapy.

Follow Up

Four to five weeks after your pellet placement, you will have follow-up blood labs to make sure that your hormones have reached the proper levels for optimal health. Up to 25% of the time, patients may need a booster shot of testosterone to reach their target levels. There is a separate fee for the booster.

Health Insurance

Unfortunately, BHRT is not covered by health insurance. However, after getting started on bio-identicals, you can expect to make far fewer trips to the doctor!

Many prospective patients say, "Dr. Brannon, I want to try this, but it costs money." And I say, "Yes, it does. But think about this: these treatments will actually benefit you for the rest of your life. Right now, and into the future. Several dollars a day is a small price to pay when compared to the cost of developing potentially life-threatening diseases later in life. Just ask any one of my patients if the cost was worth it!"

Big Pharma is opposed to BHRT because they cannot make a profit off it. Why? Because bioidentical hormones are natural. As natural products, they cannot be patented. You cannot patent an organic molecule, and therefore, the return on their investment would be extremely low in comparison to the majority of other pharmaceutical drugs - ones that they make a "killing" on.

So, at this time, health insurance typically does not cover BHRT. I don't know about you, but I don't want the government telling me how or how not to take care of myself. I don't want a bureaucrat or an insurance company telling me what type of medications I should or shouldn't take. The most important property you own is you. The one who cares the most about you is YOU.

I believe in personal liberty. And there is a freedom in taking personal responsibility for yourself.

Chapter 11 – The Pellet Placement Procedure

In this chapter, I will go into a little more detail about the pellet placement procedure, which is the part of bio-identical hormone replacement that seems to cause the most trepidation in those considering this therapy. It is really a very quick, simple, and safe procedure that most of my patients get used to in no time at all.

Pellet Placements are performed in my office every 4 to 6 months. The majority of my patients receive new pellets every 4 months. However, this is a general estimate, as the time span between placements varies from person to person. How fast you metabolize your pellets is dependent upon age, weight, ratio of body fat to muscle mass, diet, how often and how intensely you exercise, and your metabolic rate. Those that have faster metabolisms will tend to absorb the pellets a bit quicker and need pellet placements slightly more often, perhaps every three months. Once we start regularly checking your bloodwork and doing your pellet placements, we will naturally discover the optimal schedule for you to keep you feeling your best at all times.

The pellet placements are performed in The Youth Institute clinics during regular business hours Monday to Friday. You will be seen in the privacy of one of our comfortable exam rooms, where we will have the opportunity to talk briefly and address any new questions you might have.

Your appointment time will last 15 minutes. The pellet placement itself takes only 5 minutes. You may remain fully clothed. Only the area that needs to be treated will be exposed. It is best to wear sweatpants or something comfortable. You will be asked to lie down on your side and the hip area where the pellets will be inserted will be covered with a sterile drape sheet.

Placement involves a simple, sterile incision into the fatty area of one side of the buttocks. After cleaning the area with betadine and alcohol, the incision site is numbed with a 2% lidocaine solution.

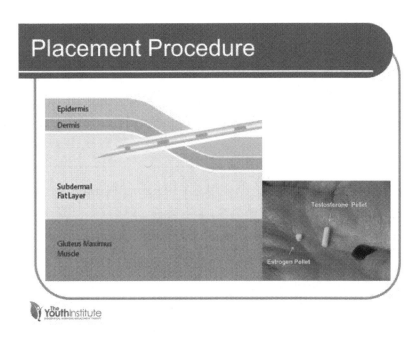

A small, straw-like instrument called a trocar is inserted at a 30-degree angle and the pellets are inserted into the fattiest part of the tissue, approximately one inch under the skin. This part of the procedure is virtually painless, because the area has been numbed. The incision is closed with steri-strip tape, then covered with tegaderm, and finally, a sterile pressure bandage. The only part of the procedure you will feel is the insertion of the needle containing the anesthetic, which is not completely painless, but most of my patients experience only minor discomfort. Very few people stop pellet therapy because of the pain of the needle!

Post-Procedure Instructions

Patients should abstain from vigorous exercise for 5 days after a pellet placement. It is normal to have swelling for 1 - 5 days and the incision may be slightly sore or itchy for up to 2 weeks afterward. There will be a bruise around the incision, which usually takes 1 - 3 weeks to fade completely. All this is normal. Your pellets can not be removed for any reason. As with any incision, there is a minimal risk of infection. This is very rare, but if it occurs, we will prescribe an oral antibiotic.

The Youth Institute Pellet

We take pride in offering you the purest type of pellet possible. Over the years, we have worked with compounding pharmaceutical companies that produce the best and most effective pellets money can buy. We use organic yams as the primary ingredient from which the testosterone is made. The pellet is 99.5% pure yam-hormone. The other 0.5% of the pellet is steric acid, which acts as a lubricant, holding the pellet together in proper form. It is important to note that the steric acid is never absorbed into your system. We don't want the pellet to be too hard, otherwise, it won't dissolve. And we don't want it to be too soft, or it won't hold together. The steric acid allows the pellet to dissolve at the optimal rate.

Typically, a man will receive anywhere from 6 to 12 pellets at a time, depending on his lab levels. His pellets will contain bio-identical testosterone, with each pellet having a dosage of 200 mg. His total testosterone dosage, per placement, will range between 1,200 and

2,400 mg. The dosage amount is based upon a precise mathematical algorithm that is individualized for every person.

The pellets we use for women contain bio-identical testosterone and estrogen. Depending on their lab work, all our female patients receive somewhere between 75 to 150 mg. of testosterone, and somewhere between 6 and 25 mg. of estrogen. In certain cases, if women are still ovulating, or have a tendency toward estrogen dominance, they may receive no estrogen at all. Each patient's case is evaluated carefully to determine what is the best course of action for her as an individual.

Pellet Expulsion

The standard literature about this procedure estimates that approximately 5 - 10% of men will expel one or more pellets per procedure. For women, the rate is much less - about 1 in 1,000. These statistics are influenced by many factors, including how hard the pellets are, what your body fat percentage is, and how high your level of physical activity is the first few days after receiving your pellets.

We try and minimize the rate of expulsion as much as possible. We're proud of the fact that our accidental expulsion rate at The Youth Institute is only **2% for men and .1% for women**. Nationally, this rate is significantly higher, but because of the high quality of the pellets we use, and also the technique of placement, we are seeing an extremely low expulsion rate.

If one or more of your pellets are expelled, you will see the pellet when you remove your bandage. It will look like a tiny, white cylindrical object, similar to a long grain of white rice. It is a good idea always to remove your bandage carefully and check for any expulsions. You will need to look closely.

So, what happens if that occurs? You simply call our office, come back in, and we will re-insert a replacement pellet. It's relatively easy.

To avoid expelling your pellets in the first place, we recommend that you refrain from vigorous physical activity, particularly on the first day, but also up to 5 days after your placement, so that your incision has a chance to heal. Try to relax and put your feet up. Read a book. Watch a movie or two. Avoid lots of walking and heavy lifting. Under no circumstances should you run, do squats, or deep knee bends.

If you have very little body fat, you will have a higher likelihood of expelling your pellets, so **lean individuals should be extra careful** during this time. If the area the pellet is placed in has a good amount of fat to cushion and surround it, there is only a small chance of expulsion. This is why, on average, women retain their pellets better. If the area around the gluteus maximus is hard with very little fat, the pellets are more easily pushed out if that muscle is contracted, which is why men have a higher rate of expulsion. This, coupled with the fact that men always receive more pellets than women do, increases the expulsion rate. So, it is primarily my male patients who will need to slow down and take it easy for the first few days after their placements.

Chapter 12 – Side Effects of BHRT

While it's true that bio-identical hormones are often described as "miraculous" because of all of the problems, disorders, and illnesses they can treat and improve, it is important to inject a dose of reality here. Bio-identical hormones are gentle, natural products which, ironically, have quite powerful effects. However, BHRT is not a cure-all. It returns your hormones to the best or most favorable levels for YOUR body, so that your body can function the way it should. You will still age, but you will age gracefully, as you were designed to. It is about giving your body an "internal advantage" to help cope with growing older.

Secondly, although there is currently no research that shows any life-threatening or long-term dangers from this therapy, there are some minor side effects of which I want all of my patients to be aware. Pellets are typically very well-tolerated. Many of these side effects will occur in the first month while the body is adjusting to the new hormone levels, but then diminish over time.

Be aware, not all patients will experience these side effects. Some patients may experience none of the following. Some may only experience one or two. However, in the spirit of full disclosure, we list every possible side effect of hormone replacement therapy so that you, the patient are able to fully weigh the risks vs. the benefits.

1. Minor Pain During Pellet Placement

There can be some minor pain for my patients during the pellet placement procedure, which happens once every three to four months. Typically, this pain lasts only a few seconds while injecting the lidocaine. It feels very similar to a bee sting. It's nobody's favorite part of BHRT, but the majority of my patients do not consider this pain a reason to stop treatment. The actual pellet insertion is nearly painless, though you may feel a slight pressure.

Some people ask, "How much pain are we talking about here?" Obviously, it differs from patient to patient, based on their level of pain tolerance. Most patients say there was "not too much pain" or "about as much as getting my blood drawn." In my experience, women have less pain, mainly because they usually receive only one pellet at a time. Whereas men can receive 6 - 12 pellets at a time, depending on their blood levels.

2. Minimal Hair Thinning or Loss

About 5 - 7% of my patients (both men and women) experience some hair thinning.

About 2 – 4% of my patients have experienced minimal amounts of hair loss.

Unfortunately, some people will experience one of these two side effects on testosterone supplementation. If either of these occurs for you, there are steps that we can take to minimize it in the future.

We recommend **biotin b7** and the herbal supplement **saw palmetto** as effective hair loss remedies. We also sell an excellent Metagenics product in our office called **Collagenics** - another alternative for hair loss prevention that works well.

3. Mild Acne

Another 1 - 3% of my patients have experienced mild break-outs of acne. This is treatable with over-the-counter acne medications and is not a long-term issue. Usually, acne will lessen over time with continued treatments. Those who experience this side effect sometimes say they don't mind breaking out like a teenager, because they also have the energy, stamina, and sex drive of a teenager!

4. Minor Facial Hair Growth

Testosterone can sometimes stimulate facial hair growth. This is not something that bothers the men, nor do they even notice, but for the 2 – 5 % of women it affects, it can be bothersome.

There are several options for solving this problem, including **electrolysis**, **waxing**, **laser hair removal**, **bleaching**, **shaving**, or a medication called **Spirolactone**, which blocks skin 5 alpha-reductase and can thin the hair. If you happen to experience this particular side effect, we can discuss which option is best for you.

5. Breast Tenderness for Women

Women who receive estrogen may experience breast tenderness, breast enlargement, or fluid retention, exactly as they would during the ovulation phase of their menstrual cycle.

Occasionally, men may experience breast tenderness as well.

We recommend evening oil of primrose to treat this symptom.

6. An Enlarged Clitoris

A small percentage of women will experience a *slight* enlargement of their clitoris. I have found that some women like it, some don't mind one way or the other, and some are unhappy with this side effect. A slightly larger clitoris is due to the testosterone supplementation. For some women, the clitoris will shrink back to its original size with continued pellet therapy, and for others, it will remain a slightly larger size. The important thing to note is that it *will not continue to grow* after its first initial "growth spurt" during the first month or two. It will remain the same size as you continue with the therapy through the years.

7. Voice Deepening

Some women or men may experience a *slight* voice deepening as a result of the testosterone therapy. This is so subtle that it is usually not noticeable to anyone but the patient.

8. Low Sperm Counts for Men

Testosterone therapy suppresses the development of sperm, therefore it is not recommended for men who are trying to conceive with a partner. Current research shows that sperm counts return to normal after pellet therapy is discontinued, should the patient decide to have children. BHRT should not, under any circumstances, be used as a method of contraception. A man will still have viable sperm on BHRT, just not as many.

9. A Decrease in Testicular Size for Men

Testosterone suppresses natural testosterone production in the testes. BHRT, in essence, does the work *for* your body, so over time, this could result in a decrease in the size of a man's testicles. This is reversible. If and when BHRT is discontinued, the testicles will return to their previous size. For most men, this is not an issue, but it's a side effect we'd like you to be aware of.

10. Higher Red Blood Cell Counts for Men

Men who are given bio-identical testosterone will experience increases in strength and energy levels. This is partly due to a proliferation of red blood cells and the extra hemoglobin that carries oxygen to all the cells in greater numbers.

Critics of BHRT speculate that an elevated red blood cell mass increases the risk of blood clots and strokes. This fear is unfounded as professional athletes whose hemoglobin counts are as high as 24 grams per deciliter do not experience cardiovascular events.[lii] However, as a precautionary measure, on the occasions when a patient's red blood cell count becomes elevated, we resolve this issue by either decreasing his testosterone a little, or recommending that he donate blood about every 4 months. Simply donating blood will allow his red blood cell count to return to normal.

11. Breast Enlargement for Men

In male patients, the body will naturally convert excess testosterone to estrogen, which can result in growth of the fatty tissue around the pectoral muscles, also known as "Gynecomastia." To avoid this, we recommend that all of our male patients take Meta I3C by Metagenics. This supplement helps metabolize excess estrogen, and for most men, it is quite sufficient. However, a few patients may require a prescription medication called Letrozole. This is an aromatase inhibitor that we use "off label" for the purpose of estrogen control.

~~~~~~

If any of these side effects sounds to you like something that would outweigh the benefits of BHRT, then I would advise you to do some additional research and take more time with your decision. **Informed Consent** is a very important part of our practice. This means that we will make every effort to be sure the patient understands the purpose, benefits, and risks of pellet therapy ahead of time. We will endeavor to make sure the patient is well-educated, with the information presented both orally and in writing. That is the foundation of ethical medicine.

Let me reemphasize that these side effects are mild, because we keep your hormones at the correct physiological levels. When you compare them to the far more serious side effects that accompany synthetic hormone treatments (high cholesterol, obesity, heart attacks, strokes, dementia, cancer, and other diseases that bio-identical hormones prevent), it is easy to see why so many people are choosing BHRT.

Who Should Not Take Bio-identical Hormones?

Pellets are not recommended for the following people:

1. Patients who have a yam allergy.

2. Women who are pregnant or wish to become pregnant within 3 months. Or, men who wish to impregnate their partner within 3 months.

3. Any person who currently has cancer or who has been treated for cancer within the last 5 years, particularly breast, uterine, or prostate cancers.

The bottom line? Bio-identicals offer incredible benefits, pose no significant health dangers, and have mild and/or infrequent side effects. They are completely natural, definitely safer, and more effective than synthetic hormones.

Chapter 13 – Common Misconceptions

There are a few common misconceptions about bio-identical hormone replacement therapy. Namely, that hormone replacement is bad for your heart, that testosterone supplementation causes prostate cancer, and that over-the-counter supplements are "the same thing" as bio-identicals. All these assumptions are false. I will address each one individually.

Fact: Bio-identical Hormones Improve Cardiovascular Function

Many of my patients have questions about their heart. There is a widespread misconception that patients with cardiovascular issues get worse with hormone treatment. That has been proven false. In fact, the reality is just the opposite. In 2000, a team of doctors at Royal Liverpool University Hospital in the U.K study discovered that treating angina patients with testosterone helped improve their condition.[liii]

In 2010, a study was published in The Journal of the American College of Cardiology that examined the effect of testosterone on people who had exercise ischemia. Exercise ischemia is a common condition whereby a person experiences an inadequate blood flow to the heart during exercise. It generally results in shortness of breath, an elevated heart rate, fatigue, and sometimes nausea and chest pain. During the study, the subjects were carefully monitored on a treadmill. At the onset of their symptoms, they were given gel-testosterone. They were not given pellets because researchers wanted to be able to see if there was an instant effect. All of the subjects felt an immediate improvement and were able to continue exercising.[liv]

A prevailing myth in the conventional medical community is that it is dangerous to give testosterone to people with bad hearts. In 2004, a study was conducted in the Department of Cardiology at Royal Hallamshire Hospital in the U.K. The researchers concluded that increased levels of bio-identical testosterone actually decreased the load on the heart. Not only were there no negative effects of administering testosterone, there were actually positive effects.[lv]

Despite the prevailing myth, studies show that hormone replacement therapy actually improves cardiovascular function.[lvi]

Fact: Testosterone Does Not Cause Prostate Cancer

One of the concerns that many men have is that hormone replacement will increase their chances of getting prostate cancer. In 2000, Dr. J.E. Morley, of The Education and Clinical Center at St. Louis V.A. Medical Center, conducted extensive research on this very subject. He concluded that, "There is no clinical evidence that the risk of either prostate cancer or benign prostate hyperplasia increases with testosterone replacement therapy."[lvii]

In 2008, The Journal of the National Cancer Institute detailed a collaborative study, combining 17 independent studies investigating the possible link between BHRT and cancer. In the end, it was surmised that, "There is no association of increased risk of prostate cancer with increased testosterone or its by-products, DHT or estradiol."[lviii]

Dr. Abraham Morgentaler is a Harvard-trained urologist and an internationally recognized expert in sexual medicine and male hormones. He wrote the phenomenal book *Testosterone for Life*. In that book, he addresses the ordinary misconception that all hormone treatments cause cancer. He published some fascinating facts. Morgentaler attacks and debunks a flawed hypothesis, put forth in 1941 by Dr. Charles Huggins. Seventy years ago, Huggins decided that testosterone increased the risk of prostate cancer, and the mainstream medical community has held his word as gospel ever since. Morgentaler took it upon himself to reread Huggins' papers, and discovered that, Huggins initially did his study on dogs, not humans! Huggins did a later study on only three men. Two of the individuals were taken off the protocol in the middle of the study, leaving only one remaining man, from which Huggins drew his conclusion. And this one subject was a castrated man! It is critical to note that all of the subsequent literature, which purports that testosterone causes prostate cancer, can be linked back to this one study. Morgentaler realized that Huggins' scientific methodology was so ludicrously inadequate that this erroneous theory "was based on almost nothing at all."[lix]

Morgentaler now has thousands of patients in his practice. In a 20-year study featured in The Journal of Urology, he documented 13 patients with biopsied prostate cancer. 30 months later, after treating them with testosterone, he biopsied them again. 54% of those patients had no residual cancer. It was gone! And the other 46% had zero increased progression or metastasis of their cancer. Morgantaler's conclusion was that, if you HAVE cancer, you actually have a 54% chance of curing it by treating it with testosterone! Additionally, you will also minimize other risks, such as cardiovascular disease and dementia.[lx]

"There is not now, nor has there ever been, a scientific basis for the belief that testosterone causes prostate cancer to grow."

~ Dr. Abraham Morgentaler[lxi]

Fact: BHRT Does Not Cause Any Type of Cancer

As a side note, let me say that there are articles all over the internet claiming that all hormone treatments cause cancer. But as I said earlier, this conclusion is based on the fact that the researchers in question have lumped all hormone treatments, synthetic and bio-identical, together. BHRT has become "guilty by association." However, I cannot find a single research paper that shows a link to cancer and bio-identicals. If there was a link between cancer and bio-identicals, you can bet that Big Pharma would have found it, and spent millions of dollars exploiting that information. Bio-identicals are a skyrocketing market, and the ever-growing competition for their patented, expensive, synthetic hormone products. As it is, there is false information that is constantly published to create intentional confusion about and distrust of natural products like bio-identical hormones. We must be very careful these days what we read, where that information comes from, and who stands to benefit from changing public opinion.

Fact: There is No Substitute for Pellet Therapy

You've probably seen the commercials on TV for over-the-counter pills and treatments that claim to increase hormone levels. Some of them are natural, herbal supplements which may be helpful for those who cannot afford pellet therapy at this time. Some of them are synthetic hormones and should be regarded with extreme caution. Over-the-counter hormone supplements of all kinds are far cheaper than pellet therapy, so many people ask me, "Are they effective?"

My answer is, "The good ones can be somewhat effective, but to a limited extent. Studies show that the majority of herbal supplements out there are not really beneficial."

For example, let's consider a man looking to increase his testosterone. He first needs to understand is there are two kinds of testosterone in his body. You will often hear the term "total testosterone." A man's total testosterone is found in two forms: bound testosterone and free testosterone. Bound testosterone can be bound to two types of proteins: albumin and sex hormone-binding globulin (SHBG). Bound T binds tightly to the hormones testosterone, DHT, and estradiol. These proteins transport testosterone throughout the body. About 98% of testosterone is bound to one of these proteins. The other 2% is known as free testosterone and loosely bound to albumin. This total makes up only 2% of bio-available testosterone. And this is the part that over-the-counter supplements might help restore. But even if it does … it's only 2%.

The important thing to understand here is that all the workouts you do and all the over-the-counter supplements you take will not increase testosterone production in your body to truly significant levels, because it's only affecting 2% of your total T. You will still wind up with a low overall T score.

Another part of the problem with "just taking some pills" is that you won't know what your initial testosterone level is, and you'll have no way of knowing if it is actually rising with the treatment. You lack real data. At The Youth Institute, we monitor your testosterone levels, from where you start at the very beginning, and continuously record your levels throughout the treatment, so that we find the optimal level for you that makes you feel great. That doesn't happen when you buy an over-the-counter supplement.

Also, BHRT does not "force" your body to increase T production. It simply supplements it. BHRT does the work for your body. It brings your levels back to where they should be and keeps them there. That's real health change. That's a difference you will feel and experience.

95% of my patients who begin bio-identical hormone replacement therapy say they will stay on it for life. In fact, it is most important that you read the personal success stories of those who have had their lives transformed by BHRT. Hear from just a few of my patients in this next chapter.

Chapter 14 – Testimonials

This next section contains the written testimonials of 11 Youth Institute patients who explain how bio-identical hormone replacement has made a difference in their lives. The first 8 were composed by me with my patients' help, and the final 3 were written in the patients' own words.

1. Derek's Story[lxii]

Derek came into my office at his mother's request. She knew some friends who were patients of mine who had seen encouraging and positive results through BHRT. As a 22 year-old, Derek had struggled for years with depression, anxiety, fear, insecurity and inferiority issues. Despite treatment from doctors and psychiatrists, his symptoms were only getting worse. A top high school athlete, he was now sedentary and lethargic, and his grades dropped to rock bottom. Shockingly, he had been contemplating suicide.

After running the appropriate lab tests, I confirmed that his testosterone levels were unusually low for his age. Seeing his need, I started him on treatments at The Youth Institute. He sensed no change after 2 weeks. After 4 weeks, still there was no discernable improvement. But 6 weeks to the day after beginning treatment, he woke up that morning and declared that "everything was different." His depression lifted. His focus returned. His testosterone had finally risen back to a normal level, and Derek had his life back again. He described it like this: "It was like someone flipped a switch and the lights came back on!" He has now returned to playing college lacrosse and excelling in school.

Why did this dramatic change happen? Derek's health and well-being returned when we put his body back in balance. His hormones were optimized to normal levels for his age and he is experiencing the benefits. Simply put, at The Youth Institute, **the NEW YOU is actually the OLD YOU!**

My heart goes out to the thousands of Dereks out there who are suffering from testosterone deficiency and have lost hope. It is tragic that men and women in their 30s, 40s, 50s, 60s, and even into their 70s have been told, "You're just going to have to live with these changes to your body."

The truth is, there is something you can do about it. And you deserve to hear the truth.

2. Bridgette's Story

Bridgette was an OB/GYN patient of mine. An athlete all of her life, she worked out and trained consistently. But when she reached her forties, she noticed that the pay-off was not what it used to be. It became more difficult for her to stay in shape. She was experiencing a combination of poor results from working out, as well as increasing lethargy. She also had been suffering from debilitating migraine headaches.

Bridgette had been following a pretty strict nutritional plan of fresh vegetables and good protein, rarely eating processed foods and very few grain products for many years. She exercised frequently, changing up her routine regularly, but still was simply not achieving the results that she used to see and feel. She was frustrated, trapped on the roller coaster of not sleeping soundly, working out more often, yet not getting the results she wanted regarding her physique.

At one of her annual examinations, she shared these struggles with me. We began talking about bio-identical hormone replacement therapy. She sounded intrigued and said she needed to research and study what I was suggesting.

Now, I LOVE that type of response. I want my patients to think for themselves. I never want them to simply take my word as truth. I encourage everyone to read, study, research, speak with those who currently receive BHRT, and make a decision based on what they believe is the best choice for them.

Bridgette started the treatment and over the following months, saw much improvement in her sleep, energy level, mood and workout results. The migraines that she was accustomed to suffering through on a regular basis were virtually gone. She rarely had to take her migraine medicine. Her body was recovering faster from workouts, her cardio endurance was increasing and she was getting stronger. Her emotional health had also improved. She felt happier and more positive. Over time, she became cognizant of when the pellets were becoming depleted, as many patients do. (Usually at the 3 to 4 month mark, most of my patients can feel when it's time for another treatment.) Bridgette has completed two Spartan races in the last year and is in better shape now than she was 10 years ago.

3. Mike's Story

No one can tell the story of "health returning" better than Mike. I've known Mike for over twenty years. He was a friend and golfing buddy before he became a patient.

Mike was a former Big 10 quarterback at Northwestern. He could throw a football 60 to 65 yards. But this once stud-of-a-guy began to see his health deteriorate. He broke his right arm, ending his playing career, and had to have a cyst removed from his right hand the day before graduation. He never had the cyst on his left hand removed, and it continued to grow and spread, entrapping the nerves up his left arm to the point where his left arm was virtually paralyzed.

He graduated and went to his first job. Over the years, his arm got worse. His wife, a registered nurse, told him, "Your arm is becoming deformed. It looks like a little alligator arm."

Thirty years of pain took its toll. Mike was continually in agony. After years of playing football, Mike also suffered from stenosis of the neck and upper back. Doctors prescribed steroid shots to ease the pain. On one occasion, one of those shots temporarily paralyzed Mike. He could not feel his lower extremities for several hours. He was wheeled into the emergency room where he eventually recovered, but he never received another steroid shot ever again.

To compensate, his doctors started prescribing lots of pain pills for him. Little did he know that those pills would further reduce his testosterone levels. That put him in a clinical depression, so the doctors prescribed more pills. Only a year ago, this once-great athlete considering the possibility of going on disability. He was self-employed and could only work four hours a day, and maybe be productive for only an hour a day. By his own admission, Mike was suffering from 20 of the 23 symptoms of low testosterone we listed in Chapter 9. As he says, "I was a mess, physically, emotionally, and spiritually - in all ways."

Mike was one of my neighbors and one day we were talking about what was going on in his body. He was depressed and discouraged. To be honest, he was also desperate. As I told him about BHRT, his face lit up. And he agreed to try it.

Within weeks, Mike's body started changing. His big belly started shrinking, and soon, he had lost all his excess weight. He recovered his muscle definition, and the pain in his upper back, neck and arm went away completely. Mike likes to explain this small miracle by saying, "I'm not a doctor. I'm an engineer and a businessman. I can't explain how all this happened. I just know I love the results. All I can do is tell you that for me, it has been nothing short of life-changing. It has made every part of my life better. I was at the golf course the other day and a woman saw me and shouted out, "WOW! Those are the biggest biceps I've ever seen!"

Mike told me recently, "Before I started BHRT, I was pale. Now I'm bronze and muscular again! I call it 'Body by Brannon.'"

Mike concluded, "People wonder if high testosterone makes you angry. From my own personal experience, I can tell you that I was angry when I wasn't happy. I struggled with anger in the years before I started on BHRT. Now it's just different. I love harder. I live harder. And I enjoy life a whole lot more."

4. Carol's Story

Carol came to see me recently. Her husband was already a patient and had encouraged her to give pellets a try, hoping to improve their sexual closeness and intimacy. Carol had been on progesterone cream therapy for several years, but her hormone levels were still significantly low. She also had a major deficiency in her Vitamin D levels. Within one week after placement, she and her husband reported back to me that her sexual responsiveness and ability to become aroused had returned. Needless to say, she and her husband are both extremely happy with pellet therapy.

5. Jake's Story

What about men? How does BHRT affect their sexual performance? Among other symptoms men often experience when their testosterone is low, Jake was suffering from erectile dysfunction. I could tell he was initially embarrassed to even bring this up with me in our consultation. I make it a point to create a safe, open atmosphere during my consultations, and Jake responded with candor. He said, "I just can't get it up like I used to. I want to have sex with my wife, but I can't get hard enough."

Once we ran his labs, it was obvious what the problem was. His testosterone was very low, which, in my office, is an easy fix! And his response was, "Doc, if you can find the solution for this, I'm all in."

After his first placement, not only did Jake see significant improvement in his ability to maintain an erection, but there were also other areas where he saw change and positive results. His energy level and ability to wake up rested and refreshed were, in his words, "back to what it used to be." In a matter of weeks, Jake was feeling like himself again.

6. Kimberly's Story

Kimberly is a 49 year-old OB/GYN patient. I've known her for many years and delivered her babies. She started pellet therapy several years ago and came in for a check-up recently. During her visit, she thanked me and said, "Over the last two years, my husband and I have finally realized what our bodies are for. Even when we were younger, we only had sexual intercourse once or twice a month. Now we are having sex 2 or 3 times a week. It's been a great way for us to communicate and draw closer as a couple. You gave us our love relationship back. You allowed me to know my body. The last several years have been phenomenal."

7. James' Story

James came into my office having done his research. At our original consultation, which lasted nearly 60 minutes, he was ready to sign up. His questions were all answered, and we ordered his labs. His testosterone level was 136, way below normal. Two days later, I performed his initial placement. I saw him at one of our public seminars about 6 weeks later and asked him how he was feeling. His labs now showed his T level to be over 1,100.

He said, "Yesterday, I worked 14 straight hours on 3 separate, highly intense projects. I was able to keep my focus, energy level, and momentum throughout the day. My thinking was clear. My spirit was energized. And I was effective. I could not have done that 6 weeks ago. BHRT is really making a difference."

Do you know what my best argument for BHRT really is? The testimonials of people like James, who have experienced dramatic changes in their lives. That's my greatest privilege – to be a part of helping bring about that change. Our goal at The Youth Institute is simply to help bring back "the old you."

8. Gary's Story

Out of all of my patients, Gary's story might be the most remarkable, because the changes to his health were so unexpected. Gary is a retired Special Agent of the U.S. Office of Personnel Management.

Gary went to see his eye doctor in Dunn, North Carolina for a routine eye exam. He was immediately referred to Dr. Overman[lxiii] of UNC Kittner Eye Center on July 11th of 2014. Dr. Overman asked him to read the letters on a standard eye chart. It was at that moment that Gary realized that he could see the letters on the sides of the chart, but not the ones in the middle. "It was as if there was a black hole in the center of my field of vision in my left eye," said Gary. Dr. Overman diagnosed him with a rare form of macular degeneration, for which there is no known cure. The doctor admitted that, in his experience with this condition, he expected Gary's vision to deteriorate rather quickly, and that he should prepare himself to be blind by the time he was 80. He explained that the sight in Gary's left eye "would slowly darken and go black over time, like the curtain lowering in a movie theater." Dr. Overman said that he did not see the benefit of taking any type of drug or supplement. He said that the type of macular degeneration Gary had was not treatable and that the gradual decline of his sight would be irreversible. Needless to say, Gary was very distressed by this news.

Gary starting taking the supplement lutein, which is reported to be beneficial for eye health. He thought it might help to slow the progress of the disease, even if it could not cure him. Then, in April of 2016, with encouragement from his girlfriend, Gary started bio-identical pellet therapy at The Youth Institute in an effort to improve his overall health. His energy level, libido, mental clarity, and mood all improved for the better and Gary was very happy with the treatments, but what happened next was something he never expected.

During his next semi-annual visit to the eye doctor on February 23rd, 2017, Gary reported that his vision had improved dramatically, although it was somewhat distorted. Dr. Overman examined him, and to his great surprise, the photo receptors in the back of his left eye and retina were being rejuvenated! Gary explained that he had started bio-identical hormones, he had been taking the lutein, and that he had also had some good people praying for him. Gary said, "My miraculous recovery has to be the result of one of those things, or perhaps all three."

Dr. Overman was genuinely astounded. He said, "I have never seen anything like this in all my years working in Opthamology. And I specialize in macular degeneration. This just doesn't happen. I have never seen a recovery of vision in any patient who has your type of MD." Dr. Overman provided Gary with high-resolution digital images of his eye before and after treatment. The images provide clear visual proof of the changes to his eye less than 10 months after starting BHRT and lutein.

When Gary came to see me for his next pellet placement, he sat down and told me the incredible story of his restored vision and the reaction of his eye doctor. Ironically, I had just been reading an article that very day about how bio-identical hormones could possibly reverse macular degeneration and end this epidemic of blindness among older Americans.[lxiv] Currently, studies are being done to prove BHRT's effectiveness for this condition. I shared the article with Gary.

I am overjoyed that one of my patients was able to reverse his macular degeneration with the help of BHRT and I look forward to helping more people like Gary in the near future.

The final three testimonials are written in the patients' own words.

9. Lindsay's Story

"Twenty years ago, I had my first GYN appointment with Dr. Brannon. So I know him well and I have trusted him as my doctor for a long time. Then, about 5 years ago, my husband and I felt that God was calling us to live and work in East Asia. The language there is one of the most difficult to learn, and my husband and I are both in our early 50s.

"About two years into our time there, we were teaching English to college students at a university in our city. They also wanted to involve us in playing ping-pong, badminton and other Asian games. I was post-menopausal and it was at that time I started thinking how little energy I had and how tired I was. I couldn't keep up with these students we were trying to minister to. In addition, my libido was low, and 6 months before a return trip to the States, I also began experiencing pain during sexual intercourse.

"I am a registered nurse by trade, and I began looking online for help. Nothing was working, and by the time we came back in the summer of 2015, I was in tears. At my annual check-up with Dr. Brannon, I shared with him what was going on.

"He looked at me and said, 'I have the answer.' And I replied, 'I knew you would!' He called me and my husband in to The Youth Institute and we had a consultation. I am very science-driven and my husband is very research-driven. We received the information and went home to do our own research and study. We looked everything up and came to the conclusion that this is what we needed to do.

"We scheduled an appointment to have our pellets placed, and my first comment to Dr. Brannon was, 'You want to put what, where?' But because I had known him for over 20 years, I trusted him.

"On the pamphlet that Dr. Brannon gave us about the benefits of BHRT, the first benefit was increased libido. I will tell you that it was probably 2 to 3 weeks later, not even at the 6-week mark, I started feeling like I was 29 years old again – not the 58 years old that I was. I was probably driving my husband crazy at that point!

"The second benefit on that pamphlet was increased clarity. My mom, who has since passed away, suffered from dementia and Alzheimer's for the last 8 years of her life. I watched her suffer from the horrific effects of those diseases. Again, after several weeks of receiving the pellet placement, I could sense clarity and focus in my mind that I hadn't had in years.

"I also have seen better cardiovascular benefits. When we returned to East Asia, I found myself, unlike before, now being able to keep up with these college students. We need energy, and that is one of the greater benefits I've experienced."

10. John's Story

"I had talked to Dr. Brannon for many years about hormone therapy. Honestly, I think the reason I didn't jump in to BHRT was ego. I work in construction. I've always been a 'man's man,' and I didn't think I needed testosterone. Whatever issues I had physically, I thought I could overcome them on my own. I think there are probably a lot of guys out there who can identify with that attitude.

"Recently, I was at a Christmas party surrounded by many who were patients of Dr. Brannon and were receiving hormone therapy. They all looked fit and trim. They had all lost weight and were in tremendous shape and they all talked so positively about it. One of those was a friend of mine who also works in construction. He's definitely someone I really respect. He's been on the hormone treatment for 3 years and finally told me, 'Dude, you just gotta do it!' And I knew it was time.

"I was convinced. I had the pellets done the next week. I know many people do not see changes in their lives as immediately as I did, but within a week, I could sense a difference. It seemed like my body was being turned into a machine that was much more in sync with itself.

"I am 57 years old and have suffered with ADD for as long as I can remember. The first real change I noticed was that 'the fog' was lifted in my head. My job in construction requires me to do some bid work, and a bunch of take-offs (material figuring). Because I've started thinking more clearly, I can set up processes much more quickly than before. Now I am usually 2 or 3 steps ahead in my mind. The hormone therapy has helped me with my concentration ten-fold.

"It has also helped my stamina on the job site. The older I've gotten, the worse my sleep became. I would wake up in the middle of the night and not be able to get back to sleep. No more. With The Youth Institute treatment, I am now sleeping through the night again and waking up refreshed. No more dog-tired, low-energy days.

"I've also had the energy to fly through workouts and am seeing changes in my body shape and muscle tone.

"I know there are a lot of people out there – especially guys – who are hesitant to start. All I can tell you is it's been a game-changer for me. My only regret is that I waited too long to start. My challenge to guys I talk with is to give it a shot. When you look at all you have to gain, I say 'Go for it!'"

11. Johanna's Story

"In March of 2014, I was diagnosed with an autoimmune disorder called Hashimoto's Thyroiditis. This condition causes a person's own body to attack the thyroid gland. The symptoms include joint pain, fatigue, brain fog, digestive issues, panic attacks, insomnia, heart palpitations, and weight changes. I had all of the above and went from a size 10 to a size 2 in the space of six months. I became very, very ill and had such debilitating joint pain that most of the time I could barely walk. At times, I needed to use crutches, and sometimes even a wheelchair. I was forced to quit my job. I was so sick that I went to live with my parents for several months. I saw thirty different doctors in one year, trying to figure out how to treat my condition.

"Unfortunately, conventional medicine is of little help when it comes to treating autoimmune disorders, which respond better to natural treatments than to drugs. Finally, I had the good fortune to find a Functional Medicine Practitioner who set me on a path to healing, using nutritional supplements and a Paleo diet. I have read and researched a tremendous amount, and I have been vigilant about sticking to the diet and taking the proper supplements. After four years, I have succeeded in putting my Hashimoto's into remission and my bloodwork continually shows that everything in my body has returned to normal.

"There were a few wonderful doctors who were instrumental in my recovery, and one of them is Dr. Greg Brannon. A problem that is common with Hashimoto's patients is hormone dysfunction, which my bloodwork confirmed. A significant part of the reason why I feel so much better is that Dr. Brannon was able to correct the erratic, abnormal fluctuations of my estrogen, progesterone, and testosterone. He did this not with dangerous synthetic hormones, but with all-natural bio-identical hormones which are made from wild yams and are actually good for your body. Bio-identical hormones, along with various other helpful treatments, have taken away my pain and allowed me to heal. I am now walking well and my life is returning to normal.

"Dr. Brannon was incredibly supportive and possesses a wealth of knowledge. He gave me a book that changed my understanding of health care and how we can make ourselves healthy without drugs or surgery. Dr. Brannon inspired me to want to help other people to heal, as he has helped me. Even when I was at my lowest point, his words of encouragement confirmed that I was doing all the right things and gave me the will to persevere.

"At my most recent appointment with him, he was astounded at how well I was walking and how much progress I've made since the last time he saw me. I assured him that a huge part of my recovery had to do with the hormone treatments, and that I was so grateful for all he had done for me. He thanked me and said, 'This is why I do what I do. Because the reward is so great when I can see a tremendous change in someone like you.' He added, 'You are a walking miracle, Johanna. Don't ever forget that. And don't ever give up your fight. You have healed yourself. Conventional medicine says you can't cure Hashimoto's, but they're wrong. You are living proof of that.' I have thought of his words many times since and they always give me strength.

"Dr. Greg Brannon is a great man and a great doctor: educated, forward-thinking, compassionate and inspiring. I am lucky to be his patient, and I hope that more people like me will be able to benefit from his care."

~~~~~~~~~~~~~~

For those of you out there suffering with depression, menopausal symptoms, low testosterone, Post Traumatic Stress Disorder, autoimmune disorders, Attention Deficit Disorder, macular degeneration, fibromyalgia, hypothyroidism, and many other common conditions, BHRT can help. There Is Hope!

Chapter 15 – The Importance of Vitamin D

There are thousands of scientific studies regarding Vitamin D3, making it one of the most studied vitamins on the planet. There is no debate in the medical community that normal Vitamin D3 levels influence human health profoundly.

At The Youth Institute, we monitor more than your hormone levels. We also track Vitamin D levels, because we know that the process of achieving optimal health requires that we address nutrition as well.

What does Vitamin D3 do?

~ Vitamin D3 affects virtually every cell in your body and affects the expression of around 3,000 genes.

~ It unlocks the genetic blueprints that are stored inside our cells.

~ Vitamin D3 promotes healthy weight, blood sugar regulation, and normal blood pressure.

~ It is involved in everything from bone strength to mood, immune function, and optimal sleeping patterns.

Vitamin D3 can help with weight loss. According to a 2007 study by The Women's Health Initiative, the combination of calcium and vitamin D3 slowed postmenopausal weight gain in women who were not getting enough calcium.[lxv] We need vitamin D to help the body absorb calcium and phosphorus from our diets. These minerals are also important for healthy bones and teeth. Anyone with metabolic syndrome, hypertension, pre-diabetes, or excess weight should have their D levels checked. If you are low, you should be supplementing with a high-quality vitamin D3 to optimize your levels.

What are the symptoms of Vitamin D deficiency?

~ Fatigue

~ General muscle pain and weakness

~ Joint pain

~ Weight gain

~ High blood pressure

~ Restless sleep

~ Poor concentration

~ Headaches

~ Bladder problems

~ Constipation or diarrhea

~ Depression

As part of your initial lab tests, we will also test your levels of Vitamin D. Once your level is determined, we will recommend your appropriate daily dose of supplementation.

The two main ways of getting Vitamin D are by exposing your bare skin to sunlight, and by taking Vitamin D supplements. Most people do not get nearly enough sunlight due to their work schedules, lifestyle, and sunscreen use. The lack of UVB (Ultraviolet B) prevents our bodies from producing enough Vitamin D.

I recommend supplementing with 5,000 to 10,000 IU of Vitamin D3 per day, depending on your individual lab levels. In addition to protecting you from the deficiency symptoms listed above, D3 can decrease your risk of obesity, diabetes, heart disease, and cancer.[lxvi]

It's important to take your Vitamin D with a meal that contains some fat, and with a high-quality Vitamin K supplement for the best absorption.

A 2012 article published by the National Institute of Health revealed that the combination of low free testosterone and low Vitamin D can be a predictor of mortality in older men. The conclusion was that this combined deficiency is commonly associated with heart attacks.[lxvii] At The Youth Institute, our goal is to make sure our patients always have "plenty of D and plenty of T" to protect their health for the long term!

Chapter 16 – Treating Thyroid Problems

I am a board-certified OBGYN, which makes me an expert in female endocrinology. I've had 25 years of experience in delivering babies, and treating and advising women regarding pregnancy, sex, diet, hormonal changes, perimenopause, menopause, and related topics. Sometimes, when I run comprehensive blood labs for my new patients, I discover that they also have thyroid abnormalities, which can be related to low or fluctuating levels of testosterone, estrogen, and progesterone. Treating the root of the problem, which is usually an underactive thyroid in this case, is an important part of the equation in making these patients feel better. My goal is not just to replace hormones, but to treat the whole individual and truly restore his/her health.

What Does my Thyroid Do?

Think of your thyroid gland as the traffic controller of your entire endocrine system; the cop in the middle of a busy intersection with a whistle! Your thyroid is at the center of all the activity, signaling what gets to go where and who gets to go first! If this master gland is asleep on the job, your body is in big trouble and there is bound to be a major traffic jam, as well as a few crashes!

The thyroid gland is located in the base of your neck, just above your collarbone. It orchestrates all of your bodily functions, including: body temperature, metabolism, digestion, cholesterol levels, heart rate, breathing, muscle development, appetite, and the release of your sex hormones. Your thyroid is continually communicating with your brain, your hypothalamus, and your pituitary gland to make all of these complicated hormonal changes happen throughout the day, every single day.

The two primary hormones released by the thyroid are Triiodothyronine (T3) and Thyroxine (T4). It is crucial that T3 and T4 levels are neither too low nor too high. I like to make sure that all of my patients are in balance, and if they need a thyroid replacement hormone, I will prescribe it for them, and counsel them on the best diet and supplements to get them back to feeling energized and healthy.

As with our BHRT, we don't view the "reference range" values on lab results as optimal. This applies to our Thyroid lab analyzation as well. Listed below are our ideal results for Thyroid Testing:

TSH   1 - 1.5 uIU/mL

Free T4 > 1.1 ng/dL

Free T3 > 3.2 pg/mL

Reverse T3 < 10 ng/dL

Thyroid Peroxidase Antibody < 9 IU/mL

Thyroglobulin Antibody 0.0 – 0.9

Ferritin 90 - 100

Our Thyroid Treatment Plans

The Youth Institute offers treatment plans for 2 types of thyroid disorder:

1. Hypothyroidism: A condition in which the thyroid gland doesn't produce enough of the thyroid hormones. Symptoms include weight gain, sleeplessness, "brain fog," constipation, dry skin and hair, depression and/or anxiety, sensitivity to cold, joint pain, muscle cramps, and extreme fatigue.

2. Hashimoto's Thyroiditis: An autoimmune disorder characterized by inflammation of the thyroid gland and severe inflammation throughout the body. Symptoms are usually the same as those for hypothyroidism, although in the early stages, Hashimoto's patients sometimes experience weight loss, heart palpitations, and panic attacks.

Full treatment plans for our thyroid patients will include:

1. An initial consultation and ongoing consultations throughout treatment.

2. Comprehensive lab testing to determine the type and severity of the thyroid disorder.

3. Recommendations for a proper diet to best address the patient's individual needs.

4. Detox information to help clean and heal the body from the inside out.

5. The best possible supplements for the patient's condition will be available for purchase in our office.

6. Prescriptions for thyroid replacement hormone or other medications the patient may require.

How BHRT Can Help

Women are eight times more likely to develop thyroid disorders than men, although thyroid disorders are becoming increasingly common for men as well. According to the American Thyroid Association, an estimated 20 million people in the United States are suffering from some type of thyroid dysfunction, and more than half are unaware of it.[lxviii] A fact that is commonly overlooked by mainstream medical professionals, is that the loss of testosterone and estrogen as we age is intricately connected to thyroid problems. It naturally follows that treating patients with bio-identical hormones goes hand in hand with restoring proper thyroid function.

At The Youth Institute, our goal is to optimize your hormones so you can look and feel your best for a lifetime. The endocrine system is very complex and delicate. The key to perfect health is balancing hormones at the ideal levels, adding high-quality nutraceuticals, and adopting a healthy diet.

With appropriate lab testing, we can help you identify the specific cause of your symptoms, and design a treatment plan that best suits you as an individual. Allow us to help you feel better than you ever dreamed possible – at any age! No, you do not have to resign yourself to feeling tired, achy, and "old." Join the thousands of men and women who have realized that with proper hormone replacement, age is truly just a number!

Chapter 17 – Conclusion and Additional Reading

I sincerely hope that I have honestly and forthrightly answered all your questions about Bio-identical Hormone Replacement Therapy. If you have more questions, I encourage you to schedule a consultation with me at one of my four North Carolina clinics so that I can give you my undivided attention.

My hope is that you now understand how hormones work in your body and why you need them to be at optimal levels.

I trust you understand the critical and life-changing difference between the synthetic hormones that Big Pharma is pushing today, and natural, safe bio-identical hormones.

I assure you, as a doctor who has studied hormones his whole life, and as a current patient receiving BHRT, this therapy will restore energy and vitality, and will keep your body youthful and healthy, able guard against various diseases as time goes on.

I have devoted the last few years of my life to making sure that The Youth Institute's pellets are the purest and best bio-identical products available today. I hope you will now take the next step and become one of my patients.

Suggested Reading

Throughout this book, I have encouraged you to do your own research. Don't simply believe what your family physician tells you. Don't believe what you hear on TV or advertisements. And don't even believe me, simply because I've said it. Take the time to investigate the topic using multiple sources and make an informed decision. Below, I recommend five key books that explain why bio-identical hormone replacement therapy is safe, proven, and effective. Check them out! All 5 of these books make reference to hundreds of articles, white papers and research studies that have been done over the years.

1. *Testosterone for Life: Recharge Your Vitality, Sex Drive, Muscle Mass and Overall Health!*, By Abraham Morgentaler, M.D.

2. *Hormone Optimization in Preventive/Regenerative Medicine*, By Ron Rothenberg, M.D.

3. *The Youth Effect: A Hormone Therapy Revolution*, By Ronald L. Brown, M.D.

4. *Feel Younger, Stronger, Sexier: The Truth About Bio-Identical Hormones*, By Dan Hale, M.D.

5. *You Don't Have to Live With It! Uncovering Nature's Power with SottoPelle Bio-Identical Hormones*, By Gino Tutera, M.D., F.A.C.O.G.

For your convenience, many of the articles mentioned in the books above are also listed on our website, which is continually updated and expanded.

You will be able to find them at:

www.youthinstitutebhrt.com

Contact Us

I began this book with you in mind - as if we were engaging in a conversation in my office. I hope this book has answered your questions. I've shown you how you can prolong Youth, Health and Vitality with Bio-identical Hormone Replacement Therapy.

The next step is up to you!

I look forward to meeting you personally and helping you get your life back. I will take great joy and pride in helping "the new you" become "the old you." (and maybe even better!)

Regardless, I would like to help you become the healthiest you that you can be.

~

Give us a call at any one of our 4 office locations:

Cary: 919-977-3231

Wake Forest: 919-727-1960

Wilmington: 910-275-4449

Southern Pines/Pinehurst: 910-377-6650

Or, call the General Information Number at:

866-789-2478

~

We look forward to helping you Stay "Forever Young!"

End Notes

---

[i] Arthur Schopenhauer, as quoted in *The Philosophical Basis of the Conflict Between Liberty and Statism*, by Donald W. Miller Jr., M.D.

[ii] Thomas Jefferson Encyclopedia, https://www.monticello.org/site/jefferson/if-people-let-government-decide-what-foods-they-eat-and-what-medicines-they

[iii] 2016 Alzheimer's Disease Facts and Figures, Alzheimer's Association

https://www.alz.org/documents_custom/2016-facts-and-figures.pdf

[iv] Heart Disease and Stroke Statistics—2017 Update: A Report From the American Heart Association

http://circ.ahajournals.org/content/early/2017/01/25/CIR.0000000000000485

[v] U.S. National Library of Medicine, The National Institute of Health, "Epigenetics: The Science of Change," by Bob Weinhold

https://www.ncbi.nlm.nih.gov/pmc/articles/PMC1392256/

[vi] Travison, T.B., A.B. Araujo, A.B. O'Donnell, V. Kupelian, J.B. McKinlay, (2007) "A population-level decline in serum testosterone levels in American men." Journal of Endocrinology and Metabolism 92:196-202.

[vii] World Health Organization, http://www.who.int/ceh/risks/cehemerging2/en/

viii Women's International Pharmacy, "A Lifetime of Progesterone."

https://www.womensinternational.com/portfolio-items/progesterone/

ix Healthy Stuff, "Phthalates: Toxic Chemicals in Vinyl Plastic."

https://www.ecocenter.org/healthy-stuff/reports/vinyl-floor-tiles/flooring_phthalate_hazards

x Williams, Graeme P., "The role of oestrogen in the pathogenesis of obesity, type 2 diabetes, breast cancer and prostate disease." European Journal of Cancer Prevention: July 2010 - Volume 19 - Issue 4 – pgs. 256-271

xi The Environmental Working Group, "Dirty Dozen Endocrine Disruptors: 12 Hormone-Altering Chemicals and How to Avoid Them."

https://www.ewg.org/research/dirty-dozen-list-endocrine-disruptors

xii Ibid

xiii Kathleen Doheny, "Statins May Lower Testosterone, Libido." WebMD

https://www.webmd.com/erectile-dysfunction/news/20100416/statins_may_lower_testosterone_libido#1

J.I. Sayer, Green Med Info, http://www.greenmedinfo.com/blog/do-cholesterol-drugs-have-men-their-gonads

xiv Lean, Michael E.J., TeMorenga, Lisa, "Sugar and Type 2 Diabetes." British Medical Bulletin, Volume 120, Issue 1, December 2016, Pages 43–53

xv Mercola, Joseph, M.D., "What Happens to Your Body When You Eat Too Much Sugar?" https://articles.mercola.com/sugar-side-effects.aspx

xvi Nordqvist, Christian, "How does Bisphenol A affect health?" Medical News Today, https://www.medicalnewstoday.com/articles/221205.php

xvii Michael J. Breus, M.D., "Testosterone, Sleep And Sexual Health," Huffpost (2011), https://www.huffingtonpost.com/dr-michael-j-breus/testosterone-sleep-sexual-health_b_981121.html

xviii Sanders, Robert, "Pesticide Atrazine can turn male frogs into females." U.C Berkley (2010), http://news.berkeley.edu/2010/03/01/frogs/

xix EcoWatch, Organic Consumers Association, "Glyphosate Found in Urine of 93 Percent of Americans Tested." May 29th, 2016

https://www.ecowatch.com/glyphosate-found-in-urine-of-93-percent-of-americans-tested-1891146755.html

xx Neil Z. Miller, Gary S. Goldman, "Infant mortality rates regressed against number of vaccine doses routinely given: Is there a biochemical or synergistic toxicity?" Human & Experimental Toxicology, (2011) 30(9): 1420–1428.

xxi Joseph Mercola, M.D., "Vaccines Have Serious Side Effects - The Institute of Medicine Says So!"

https://articles.mercola.com/sites/articles/archive/2011/09/27/vaccines-are-dangerous-says-the-government.aspx

[xxii] Pam Harrison, "Low Vitamin D Tied to Testosterone Dip in Healthy Men." May 27, 2015, Medscape https://www.medscape.com/viewarticle/845483

[xxiii] Michael Connett, "Tooth Decay Trends in Fluoridated vs. Unfluoridated Countries." Fluoride Action Network, July 2012.

http://fluoridealert.org/studies/caries01/

[xxiv] Edward Group DC, NP, DACBN, DCBCN, DABFM, "9 Shocking Dangers of Fluoride Exposure," November 16, 2015, Global Healing Center

https://www.globalhealingcenter.com/natural-health/9-shocking-dangers-of-fluoride/

[xxv] Molly M. Shores, MD; Alvin M. Matsumoto, MD; Kevin L. Sloan, MD; et al, "Low Serum Testosterone and Mortality in Male Veterans," August 14, 2006, The Journal of the American Medical Association.

https://jamanetwork.com/journals/jamainternalmedicine/fullarticle/410768

[xxvi] Khaw, K.T., Dowsett, M., Folkerd, E., et al. "Endogenous testosterone and mortality due to all causes, cardiovascular disease, and cancer in men: European prospective investigation into cancer in Norfolk (EPIC-Norfolk) Prospective Population Study." Circulation 2007; 116 (23): 2694-2701.

[xxvii] Korenman, S.G., Morley, J.E., Mooradian, A.D., et al. (1990) "Secondary hypogonadism in older men: its relationship to impotence." The Journal of Clinical Endocrinology and Metabolism 71:963-969.

[xxviii] Shores, M.M., Matsumoto, A.M., Sloan, K.L., Kivlahan, D.R. "Low serum

testosterone and mortality in male veterans." JAMA Internal Medicine 2006; 166 (15): 1660-1665.

xxix Hak, A.E., Witteman, J.C., DeJong, F.H., et al. "Low levels of endogenous androgens increase the risk of arthrosclerosis in elderly men: the Rotterdam study." The Journal of Clinical Endocriniology and Metabolism 2002, 87:3632-9.

xxx *Testosterone For Life*, by Abraham Morgentaler, M.D., McGraw Hill, copyright 2009, page 53.

xxxi O. Johnell, J.A. Kanis, "An estimate of the worldwide prevalence and disability associated with osteoporotic fractures." (2006) Osteoporosis International 17:1726.

xxxii J.A. Kanis, World Health Organization Technical Report 2007, University of Sheffield, U.K.:66.

xxxiii The European Foundation for Osteoporosis and Bone Disease, National Osteoporosis Foundation (1997) "Who are candidates for prevention and treatment of Osteoporosis?" Osteoporosis International 7:1.

xxxiv O. Johnell, J.A. Kanis, Ibid, Osteoporosis International 17:1726.

xxxv L.J. Melton the 3rd, E.J. Atkinson, M.K. O'Connor, et al. (1998) "Bone density and Fracture Risk in Men." Journal of Bone and Mineral Research 13:1915; L.J. Melton the 3rd, E.A. Chrischilles, C. Cooper, et al. (1992) "Perspective: How Many Women have Osteoporosis?" Journal of Bone and Mineral Research 7:1005; J.A. Kanis, O. Johnell, A. Oden, et al. (2000) "Long-term Risk of Osteoporotic Fracture in Malmo." Osteoporosis International 11:669.

xxxvi J.W.W. Studd, et al. (1990) American Journal of Obstetrics and Gynecology 163:1474 – 1479: Christiansen, et al. (1981); Lindsay, et al. (1976); Stevenson, et al. (1990).

xxxvii Dorgan, J.F., Albanes, D., Taylor, P.R., et al, "Endogenous sex hormones and prostate cancer: a collaborative analysis of 18 prospective studies," February 6, 2008, Journal of the National Cancer Institute.

https://www.ncbi.nlm.nih.gov/pubmed/18230794

xxxviii Julia A. Files, M.D., Marcia G. Ko, M.D., Sandhya Pruthi, M.D., "Bio-identical Hormone Therapy." Mayo Clinic Proceedings, July 2011, Volume 86, Issue 7, Pages 673–680.

xxxix The Hormone Solution, Stay Younger Longer with Natural Hormone and Nutrition Therapies by Thierry Hertoghe, M.D., Copyright 2002, Three Rivers Press.

xl A. Fournier, F. Berrino, E. Riboli, V. Avenel, F. Clavel-Chapelon, "Breast cancer risk in relation to different types of hormone replacement therapy in the E3N-EPIC cohort." International Journal of Cancer, 2005; 114:448–454.

xli "Natural vs. Organic," taken from the website: Organic. It's Worth It., May 30, 2018.

http://www.organicitsworthit.org/natural/natural-vs-organic

xlii John P. Cunha, DO, FACOEP, "side Effects of Premarin," October 17, 2016, RX List.

https://www.rxlist.com/premarin-side-effects-drug-center.htm#overview

xliii Omudhome Ogbru, PharmD, "Side Effects of Provera," September 13, 2016, RX List. https://www.rxlist.com/provera-side-effects-drug-center.htm

xliv Wendy Y. Chen, MPH, MD, "Postmenopausal Hormone Therapy and Breast Cancer Risk: Current Status and Unanswered Questions," July 12, 2011, The National Institute of Health. https://www.ncbi.nlm.nih.gov/pmc/articles/PMC3167091/

xlv Craig, M.C., Maki, P.M., Murphy, D.G., "The Women's Health Initiative Memory Study: findings and implications for treatment," March 2005, The National Institute of Health. https://www.ncbi.nlm.nih.gov/pubmed/15721829

xlvi A. Fournier, Ibid. 114:448-454

xlvii A. Fournier, Ibid. 114:448-454

xlviii Tang, M.X., Jacobs, D., Stern, Y., Marder, K., Schofield, P., Gurland, B. (1996) "Effect of estrogen during menopause on risk and age at onset of Alzheimer's disease." Lancet 348:429–432.

xlix Gouras, G.K. et al. Proceedings of the National Academy of Sciences of the United States of America USA, (2000) 97(3):1202-5; Tan, R.S., "A pilot study on the effects of testosterone in hypogonadal aging male patients with Alzheimer's disease." Aging Male (2003); 6(1):13-7.

l Thomas G. Travison Andre B. Araujo Amy B. O'Donnell Varant Kupelian John B. McKinlay, "A Population-Level Decline in Serum Testosterone Levels in American Men," The Journal of Clinical Endocrinology & Metabolism, Volume 92, Issue 1, January 2007, Pages 196–202 li Erlingur Nordal, "Testosterone levels decreasing in Danish men," May 17, 2010, IceNews.

http://www.icenews.is/2010/05/17/testosterone-levels-decreasing-in-danish-men/#axzz4f1HF2xrr

lii Clearfield Medical Group, "Bioidentical Hormone Replacement Therapy (BHRT) for Men," taken from their website on May 31st, 2018. https://drclearfield.net/bhrt-for-men/

liii K.M. English, O. Mandour, R.P. Steeds, M. J. Diver, T.H. Jones and K. S. Channer, "Men with coronary artery disease have lower levels of androgens than men with normal coronary angiograms." Department of Clinical Chemistry, Royal Liverpool University Hospital, Liverpool, U.K.

liv C.J. Malkin, P.J. Pugh, P.D. Morris, K.E. Kerry, R.D. Jones, T.H. Jones, K.S. Channer, "Cardiovascular Medicine: Testosterone replacement in hypogonadal men with angina improves ischemic threshold and quality of life,." Heart 2004; 90:871-876.

lv Ibid, https://www.ncbi.nlm.nih.gov/pmc/articles/PMC1768161/

lvi Ferdinando Iellamo, M.D., Maurizio Volterrani, M.D., Guiseppe Caminiti, M.D., Roger Karam, M.D., Rosalba Massaro, M.D., Massimo Fini, M.D., Peter Collins, M.D., GiusseppeM.C. Rosano, M.D., "Testosterone Therapy in Women with Chronic Heart Failure: A Pilot Double-Blind, Randomized, Placebo-Controlled Study." The Journal of The American College of Cardiology, (2010) 56(16):1310-1316.

lvii Mayo Clinic Proceedings, Ibid, January 2000

[lviii] The Journal of The National Cancer Institute, Ibid, 2008

[lix] Morgentaler, Ibid, pages 116-128.

[lx] Morgentaler, Ibid, pages 79-93.

[lxi] Morgentaler, Ibid, page 125.

[lxii] All of the stories and testimonials presented in this book are 100% true. In some cases, I have merely changed the name of the patient to protect his/her privacy.

[lxiii] The surname of this individual has been changed to protect his/her identity.

[lxiv] Debora Yost, "Preventing Macular Degeneration: A New Theory: Pioneering Eye Surgeon Sees Hope for Treating Macular Degeneration with Natural Hormones," December 2008, Life Extension Magazine.

http://www.lifeextension.com/Magazine/2008/12/Preventing-Macular-Degeneration/Page-01

[lxv] Bette Caan, DrPH; Marian Neuhouser, PhD; Aaron Aragaki, MS; et al, "Calcium Plus Vitamin D Supplementation and the Risk of Postmenopausal Weight Gain," May 14, 2007, The Journal of The American Medical Association.

https://jamanetwork.com/journals/jamainternalmedicine/fullarticle/412368

[lxvi] Hanmin Wang, Weiwen Chen, Dongqing Li, Xiaoe Yin, Xiaode Zhang, Nancy Olsen, and Song Guo Zheng, "Vitamin D and Chronic Diseases," May 2017, Aging and

Disease. https://www.ncbi.nlm.nih.gov/pmc/articles/PMC5440113/

lxvii U.S. National Library of Medicine, National Institute of Health, "Combination of low free testosterone and low vitamin D predicts mortality in older men referred for coronary angiography." https://www.ncbi.nlm.nih.gov/pubmed/22356136

lxviii The American Thyroid Association, taken from the "General Information/Press Room" page on their website, May 30, 2018. https://www.thyroid.org/media-main/about-hypothyroidism/

Made in the USA
Columbia, SC
29 July 2019